THE NAET GUIDE BOOK

The Companion to

"SAY GOODBYE TO ILLNESS"

BY

Dr. Devi S. Nambudripad

D.C., L.Ac., R.N., O.M.D., Ph.D.

Published by

Delta Publishing Company
6714 Beach Blvd.
Buena Park, CA 90621
FAX: (714) 523-3068

DEDICATION

This book is dedicated to all the patients
who call their doctors day after day
to ask many questions
about the Nambudripad's Allergy Elimination Program.

ACKNOWLEDGEMENT

I would like to thank a few people who encouraged me to write this book. First of all, I have to acknowledge my thanks to the confused, scared, frustrated NAET patients who called me many times during my office hours and even at night on the emergency line to get their questions answered. When I received almost the same questions from every one that called, I decided to answer them in this book form. This should be read by patients and doctors. This should save some time for both parties.

My special thanks also go to my son Roy and my husband Kris and those who helped me to put my ideas into book form. I would also like to thank my printers who did a great job on printing this book.

First Edition, January 1994
Second Edition, May 1996
Third Edition, September, 1998

Copyright 1998
by
Devi S. Nambudripad, D.C., L.Ac., R.N., O.M.D., Ph.D.

Library of Congress Catalog Number: 98-93633
ISBN:0-9658242-2-5

All rights reserved

Printed in U.S.A.

PREFACE

The purpose of this book is to help practitioners who treat their patients with Nambudripad's Allergy Elimination Techniques (NAET) and the patients who undergo the NAET treatments. When the practitoners take the seminars, they seem to understand everything. But when they begin to work with allergic patients, many questions come up. Then, from their busy schedule they have to make time to contact our office or another practitioner who attended the seminar to get their questions answered. Likewise, when patients go through NAET treatments, they also have many questions. Since this is a new method of treatment, patients get confused without understanding the whole procedure. They also are frustrated when they do not get their hundreds of questions answered by their busy practitioners.

This book hopefully will answer most of your questions and help you to go through the treatments easily and happily. The "You may eat section" will help the patient have a few essential items to eat during the 25-hour period. Readers should understand that this list does not give the complete list of food and food products allowable. It is advisable to consume a minimum number of food items during the 25-hour clearing stage. This will help the body to dispense less energy for food digestion and more energy to help clear the blockages of the energy pathways.

For the best and fastest results, patients are encouraged to get treatments in the order of allergens specified in this book. Before the patients come to the practitioner's office, they can look up the next prospective item for the treatment and plan the lifestyle for the next 25 hours. This way the patients can help themselves get through the treatments with less stress.

Record-keeping is a problem for everybody. But accuracy of record keeping will help the patient to achieve maximum results in a short period of time. This book is designed to help the patient and the practitioner keep better treatment records with less effort. This book can replace the runner file in the office. Practitioners can keep one book for each patient and mark the treatments and results in the book. The patient can keep another book for himself or herself, and he/she can have a personal journal about his/her treatments.

Patients are encouraged to read "Say goodbye To Illness" prior to starting NAET treatments with their practitioner. This book will give you some understanding about allergies, allergy related diseases, and how a non-invasive, easy to follow, holistic treatment can give you freedom to live again. Many case histories of managing various health problems are given in "Say Goodbye To Illness". Young infants from day five to older patients as old as 94 have been treated with NAET with excellent results. Many so-called incurable problems have been traced to food or environmental allergies and treated with great success.

The current list of the NAET specialists who have completed the NAET Basic and Advanced training and who are qualified to treat with NAET is available from PAIN CLINIC, 6714 BEACH BLVD., BUENA PARK, CA 90621. FAX: (714) 523-3068. Also look up our website: http://www.allergy-naet.com.

If I can somehow lessen the frustration of the patients and the practitioners, and help the patients get well and lead a normal life, my dream is fulfilled.

Devi S. Nambudripad, D.C., L.Ac., R.N., O.M.D., Ph.D.

Buena Park, CA.

September, 1998

THE NAET GUIDE BOOK

COMPANION TO "SAY GOODBYE TO ILLNESS"
BY
DR. DEVI S. NAMBUDRIPAD, D.C., L.Ac., R.N., O.M.D., Ph.D.

This Guide Book has been prepared as a handy practical reference for patients as they go through the process of treatment for various allergies according to Nambudripad's Allergy Elimination Techniques (NAET). We cannot overemphasize the need for complete cooperation between the patient and the doctor in order to achieve the most satisfactory results with the least discomfort, inconvenience or complications to the patient.

All patients are expected to read the book "SAY GOODBYE TO ILLNESS" before they become NAET patients. It is very important for the patient to understand the NAET approach thoroughly before they begin their NAET treatments. This book will help you understand all about food and environmental allergies and will answer the most commonly asked questions about allergies.

Since NAET is a new development in the field of "Medicine," it is not widely known among the medical community or the public. We do not, as yet, have enough written material on NAET circulating among interested people. As people discover NAET, through friends or books, even though it is a non-invasive, gentle, allergy elimination technique, they may be anxious or fearful due to previous lack of information. My book, "Say Goodbye To Illness," will explain what NAET is all about and what it can do to improve your health. A number of actual case histories, about various allergies and allergy-related illnesses, will render the prospective patient with enough confidence and encouragement to try this new technique. <u>Lessening the patient's fear and concern about our allergy elimination treatment will make the patients' and doctors' lives easier while going through the treatment.</u> When you understand the treatment and completely cooperate with the NAET doctor, you can achieve better and faster results.

DOCTOR'S OFFICE

Let's begin our journey with the NAET practitioner's office. The NAET practitioner must take special care to keep his/her office suitable to accommodate allergic patients. When the patients find a particular practitioner's office comfortable and safe for them to be in during the few minutes' treatment, word will spread quickly through the vast allergic community (which is now one of the largest communities, worldwide). Patients will actually begin flying to that office from all over the world. So it is very important for the practitioners to keep their offices as comfortable as possible, if they are seriously going to treat allergic patients with NAET.

The office should be kept clean at all times. The practitioner should try to renovate and refurnish the office with hypoallergenic carpets, paints, chairs, etc. Chemical cleaning agents with strong smells are to be completely avoided. The office should be free from cooking smells, fragrances from flowers, soaps, incense, perspiration and body odors, massage oils, aroma therapy oils (natural, organic or synthetic), herbal extracts and oils, hair sprays, deodorants, etc. Patients with food and environmental allergies are very sensitive to mold, dust, smells from air-conditioning or heating units and vents. Smells from perfume, formaldehyde, newspaper, wall paper, Clorox, bleaches, detergents, fabric softeners, carpet deodorizers, air fresheners, old or fresh paint are devastating for environmentally sick patients. The practitioner must take special care that all of his patients and staff follow the rules correctly. No one should ever wear perfumes or scented hair sprays. Fresh flowers or plants must not be allowed in the office.

Staff and patients should be instructed not to eat food in the patient association areas. Food preparation, brewing coffee, popping popcorn, cooking in the microwave oven, etc. should be prohibited in the office. Air purifiers can be used to remove unhealthy smells from the rooms or the whole office. Electric air purifiers can sometimes cause unpleasant reactions in patients with electric or electromagnetic sensitivity. It is not advisable to use such equipment in the presence of such patients. Avoid loud music and loud noises. If there are noisy children among patients, parents can move them to another room where they can entertain themselves while waiting. Loud noises can irritate environmentally sensitive people. These immune deficient patients can faint or lose control of their equilibrium and muscles in the presence of any smell or loud noises. The receptors for smell and hearing become super sensitive in the environmentally sick person.

BUDDY SYSTEM FOR PRACTITIONERS

Practitioners should form a buddy system with other practitioners in the vicinity of their offices to encourage a support system. If a practitioner cannot find the cause of a flare up condition in a patient, or if he/she needs help with a new case, the buddy system can help. Sometimes two heads are better than one. Please do not be hesitant to ask for help if you need it. No one is perfect, and we all may need help sometimes. After all, our aim is the patient's welfare. We have more than 2000 well qualified NAET practitioners around the country. It is very easy to form small groups in your area. NAET buddy practitioners should make it a point to meet once a week or once a month, to exchange ideas and suggestions to help each other. Whenever anyone comes up with a new useful idea, please share it with Nambudripad's Allergy Elimination Group family, also known as Nambudripad's Allergy Research Foundation or "N.A R F."

CLEARING PRACTITIONER'S ALLERGIES

It is imperative that practitioners know they must clear their own allergies as soon as possible. They may have a parallel weakness to the patients' allergen. When the practitioner is free of his allergies, his energy system is balanced and refined. In that way he is more effective using muscle response testing with allergic patients. The practitioner must be proficient in his/her muscle response testing ability since NAET depends on MRT to determine allergies and plan the appropriate treatments.

NAMBUDRIPAD'S ALLERGY RESEARCH FOUNDATION OR N.A.R.F.

Our nonprofit foundation, N.A.R.F. is dedicated to further investigation and research in NAET. The Foundation sends out a bimonthly newsletter (6 issues/year) to members for a subscription fee of $36.00 per year. We publish all new developments in the field of NAET. The Foundation holds an annual NAET symposium. All trained NAET practitioners are invited to participate at the symposium to learn from one another. NARF has a web-site. NAET practitioners who have completed the advanced NAET training and have satisfied the training requirement of NARF will be listed on the site. If the practitioner would like to advertise through the site, a single page can be purchased through NARF for a nominal fee. To get information about membership to the Foundation, web-site or the newsletter, please write to:

NARF Newsletter

6732 BEACH BLVD.

BUENA PARK, CA 90621

(Phone): (714) 523-8900 / 523-3500   Fax: (714) 523-3068.

SUPPORT GROUP FOR PATIENTS

It is a good idea to form a support group for the allergic patients. Encourage the patients who are beginning to get well, and are on the way to recovery, to form a support group among themselves. With permission their telephone numbers can be made available to the newer patients. If new patients experience any unpleasant allergic reactions during treatments they can talk and give moral support to one another.

Family and friends are encouraged to get involved with the patient's treatment. Most patients suffer from unpleasant reactions while they go through the first few treatments. It is very important to maintain the patient's spirit during this time. Any support will help. If someone has no family, they should at least have a friend to help through the initial days of treatment. Some severely allergic patients can experience unpleasant reaction anywhere from few hours to 25-30 hours after the treatment. It will be comforting for the patient to talk to some supportive person during those hours. Patients' support group can help with this situation if someone doesn't have family.

NORMAL REACTION AFTER TREATMENTS

Is there a "normal" reaction after a successful NAET treatment during the first 25-hour period? Some patients experience no changes with their first NAET treatments. A few patients find the changes to be very subtle. Others may experience one or more symptoms from the list given below. Anything you notice, other than being pain-free, with an overall sense of well being mentally and physically, is a reaction. The intensity of the reactions during the first 25-hour period depends on many factors, such as the duration of the illness, intensity of the illness, and the status of the immune system.

PHYSICAL SYMPTOMS

Feeling high or low energy, extreme fatigue, tingling sensation anywhere in the body, itching of the body, hives, sensation of electricity in the body, sensation of various kinds of pain every now and then anywhere in the body like shooting pain, dull or distended pain, pin prick sensation, tightness in the chest, sensation of energy movements anywhere in the body, sensation of variation of temperature in the body, sleepiness, insomnia, restlessness, hyperacidity, abdominal bloating, belching, hiccups, sensations of dust-like particle in the lungs, sneezing, coughing, tearing, post nasal drips, palpitation, cardiac arrhythmia, increased blood pressure, decreased or increased heart rates, paroxysmal tachycardia, sudden venous congestion or varicose vein, excessive or low libido, general body ache, etc., are some of the physical symptoms experienced by allergic patients.

EMOTIONAL SYMPTOMS

Crying spells, anxiety, nervousness, fainting, anger, rage, empty feeling in the mind, butterfly sensation in the stomach, mood swings, obsession, depression, suicidal thoughts, laughing spells, numbness, blurred vision, choking, throat constriction, claustrophobia, nausea, headaches, ringing in the ear, sensations of hairlike particles in the eye, diarrhea, constipation, itching in the private areas of the body in either sex, impotency, low libido, various cravings like salt, sugar, spices, sour things, coffee, popcorn, sweet smells of flowers or perfumes, smells of chemicals like bleach, etc., smell of sweat, etc. are some of the emotional symptoms. I had a patient who carried her husband's sweaty shirt during the 25-hour period and smelled it often to keep her from getting depressed.

Most of the time, if one experiences one or more symptoms from the list of physical symptoms, NAET treatment at the spinal level is adequate along with acupressure/acupuncture at the gate points. If the patient experiences any symptoms from the list of emotional symptoms, emotional components also should be checked and treated.

Occasionally a patient may experience the symptoms immediately or within the twenty-minute waiting period in the doctor's office. If that happens, the patient is advised to inform any changes to the doctor immediately. The doctor can administer further treatments as needed before he/she leaves the office.. In some cases, it may take many hours for the patient to experience unpleasant symptoms. Some patients have gone as long as 23 ½ hours before they experienced any unpleasant symptoms. In that case the patient may have to suffer the symptoms until he or she returns to the office, unless they have been taught to balance their own body, in order to reduce or eliminate unpleasant symptoms. "LIVING PAIN FREE" with acupressure by this author may be helpful to learn self balancing techniques. This book is available at many book stores and at Delta publishing Co. (Check the resources at the back).

COMMONLY SEEN REACTIONS DURING NAET

While going through NAET, patients can respond in many ways:

Group 1. These are the patients who feel great relief immediately after their first NAET treatment and continue to feel good. They may be presently sick and allergic to many items, but have found a way to maintain a strong immune system. When the body is clean, without many toxins in the system, NAET treatments are easier and faster. It is advisable to go through some cleansing program when you suffer from severe allergic reactions. For example, taking immune system stimulants, going through some effective detoxifying programs like liver cleansing, colon cleansing with herbal products, homeopathic products; limiting the variety of food intake, juice fast, allergy shots, colonics, vigorous exercises are things to consider. Incorporating yoga and meditation practices, regular chiropractic or acupuncture treatments, enzyme therapy, vitamins, mineral or herbal supplements, etc. into one's life-style on a regular basis, will render beneficial effects.

The Liver — our garbage disposal, gets overloaded with accumulated toxins. Toxins, under pressure, will convert into heat and circulate in the body. The trapped heat will cause blockages in various parts of the energy channels giving rise to various health problems. The presenting symptoms will be directly related to the area that is being blocked. If the lung energy channel is blocked, the patient can suffer from respiratory disorders like bronchitis, asthma, etc. If the colon energy channel is blocked, the patient can suffer from constipation, diarrhea, eczema, skin disorders, etc. This unwanted heat cannot come out of the body without some help. Chiropractic manipulations, acupuncture, a liquid or water fast, exercise, sauna, cleansing programs, detoxifying programs, etc., can create a port for the trapped toxic heat to exit the body. Regularly done, any of the above programs will release the toxic heat as soon as it is produced.

Group 2. These patients may feel good soon after the treatment, however, as the hours go by they may begin to experience tiredness. Some patients can sleep through 25 hours. Some in this group can take as long as 35-40 hours to pass a treatment. When they complete the hours, this group usually feels better.

Group 3. This group of people may not feel good soon after the treatment, but as the hours go by they get better and towards 25 hours they feel great. 1 capsule of "Vitality formula" following each meal after clearing the allergy will be helpful (available from Lotus Herbs, Inc.).

Group 4. Patients from this group may experience a roller coaster effect. Initially, they may experience very slight or no improvements at all. They may have a few good hours in a day once they have gone through five to ten basic treatments. Gradually, as they receive more treatments they will have more good hours of relief. Eventually the number of good days will outnumber the bad days, until finally, they experience all good hours and days.

These patients fall into the immune deficiency disorder group, suffering from long standing chronic illnesses or a low immune system. These patients may need to be treated with many combinations.

Group 5. Patients from this group may have suffered from many emotional traumas and various types of abuses since childhood. Continuous emotional traumas may have caused the immune system to weaken. This poor immune system will lead them to physical and chemical reactions as well. As the immune system becomes weak, patients will begin to react to all substances around them. They need to be treated and cleared physically for basic allergens to strengthen their immune system. Along with the basic treatments, they should also receive emotional clearance of their traumas. Some suffer from painful flashbacks. They can even become suicidal at times. Such patients should also receive professional psychological counselling along with NAET regular treatments and NAET emotional treatments. They will need continuous emotional support for long time even after completion of NAET. NAET specialists are not trained mental health specialists (psychologists or psychiatrists). NAET specialists are trained to unblock the obstructed emotions in connections with food and environmental substances. During the NAET treatments for emotional conditions, the normal flow of energy through the emotional parts of the energy meridians will be reestablished. Because of the normal energy flow patients will feel better. But we should remember that mentally or emotionally sick people have their weaknesses in the emotional parts of the energy meridians. The emotions are also transmitted through certain physical areas of the nerve fibers. If these segments of the nerve fibers are weak, repeated reactions can affect these areas and the emotional reactions can repeatedly take place until the area gets stronger. Emotionally hypersensitive people should take nerve strengthening supplements for a long time along with emotional support (Counselling). This group will also require combination treatments with the allergen and brain tissue or different parts of brain. Please check with your practitioner for more information. These patients will need large amounts of B-Complex, minerals, and amino-acid supplements high in L-Glutamine, phenylalanine, and Tyrosine after clearing the allergy. The herbal preparation "Bupleurum and Dragon Bone formula" 1X3 after meals, is very effective in mild to moderate cases (available from Lotus Herbs, Inc.).

NAET emotional treatments are very effective when the patient shows emotional blockages along with food and other substances. There are other holistic emotional treatments patients can seek along with NAET. They are "Neuro Emotional Techniques" (NET, check the Resources at the back) and "La Chance Release Techniques". If someone suffers from severe emotional blockages, they may consider the care of a psychiatrist during this release method and, if necessary, non-allergic herbal or prescription medication should be used to control depression, severe mood swings, unpleasant or scary flashbacks. The NAET practitioner can test each supplement or medication for allergy. If necessary, the patient should be treated for the medicine before they take it. By keeping their presenting symptoms under control, they will be able to go through NAET faster and easier.

DAILY LOG

Patients are encouraged to maintain a daily log of all the different foods they are eating, any and all symptoms they are experiencing, all the places and people they are visiting. All other activities and events, especially if there is an unusual one, like a new visitor to the family, death or accidents in the family, divorce or any unhappy events, any newborn and new additions to the family are to be noted. After two or three successful NAET treatments, it is suggested they eat food from the list that they have been treated for and have passed.

WHAT IS A SUCCESSFUL NAET TREATMENT?

The patient is rechecked with MRT, (Muscle Response Testing) for the allergen 25 hours or more after the NAET treatment. The patient's indicator muscle should test very strong in the presence of the treated allergen. This strong response is called a successful treatment. For example, 25 hours after the first treatment of "Egg mix", if the indicator muscle tests very strong, we can assume that about 80-90% of the allergy to the egg mix (egg white, egg yolk and chicken) is gone and it is safe to use the product. With the first treatment to a complex food item like "egg mix", one will not get 100% freedom from that allergy. Because egg has many nutrients, it is not easy to clear all the nutrients in one treatment. The rest of the 10-20% of the allergy to the egg will clear up when they complete all the basic treatments. Some severely allergic cases may need a few more combination treatments to be able to eat egg freely.

Egg is a good protein and highly reactive item in many people. Egg contains many vitamins and minerals. NAET basic treatments treat all the essential vitamins and minerals along with the particular basic food groups. When you finish the basic treatments, the vitamin-mineral contents of the egg will also clear. With that, the rest of the 10-20% of the egg allergy will clear. If the indicator muscle tests slightly mushy, you will need to treat the egg again until you show a strong MRT since the mushy muscle-test shows that only 50-60% of the allergy is gone. You can have an allergic reaction when you eat or use products with 40-50% allergy still left in your body. After they clear the allergy with NAET (strong MRT), patients should be encouraged to eat a small portion of the food daily for few days. This way the new imprinted memory will stay strong in the brain's memory bank. After they have satisfactorily consumed the food for few times, they can add that to their daily list. After they have cleared the allergy to a few groups (about 5 groups), they should be encouraged to eat those items exclusively until they clear for more items. This way they can reduce or get relief from their presenting symptoms.

When one is highly allergic to all the nutrients in the food, it is not advisable to eat 100% organic food soon after the NAET treatments. Organic products are very nutritious and complex. It takes more energy to digest and assimilate nutrients from complex nutritious products. Initially for a few weeks or in some cases even months after the treatment, it is better to eat semi-whole grain products, for example, 50% wheat bread, etc. Fruits and vegetables should be cooked before you consume them to avoid reactions. Fruit juices can be heated first and then cooled before you drink them. Cooking helps to digest the food faster. Gradually, you can train your body to digest the wholesome foods without any adverse reactions. In some cases like Crohn's disease, irritable bowel syndrome, ulcerative colitis, etc., it may take more than a year before they can eat uncooked wholesome products without any reaction. In these cases with a weak digestive tract, it is advisable to eat well cooked, non-allergic food to avoid pain and discomfort. Small frequent meals are also suggested in these cases. Taking "Agastache formula" (Lotus Herbs, Inc.) 1 capsule 15 minutes before meals helps the digestion and "Multizyme" 1X3 after meals (Available from Standard process of so Ca).

SURROGATE TREATMENT

When the patient gets treated with NAET, patient and practitioner should be alone in the room. If the patient is unable to test and treat himself/herself, they can be treated through a surrogate.

A third person or animal in the room can steal the treatment from the patient. In such cases, the third person will get better and the patient will get sicker or show no improvement. Small children should not accompany mothers for NAET treatments. If the patient is getting tested or treated through a surrogate, the patient should maintain a constant skin-to-skin contact with the surrogate during testing and treatment. If the patient loses the contact intermittently, the treatment may not work.

Mary, a 30 year-old mother received treatment for 9 months. She was treated for over 62 items. The patient began getting worse day after day instead of getting better. Finally, the desperate practitioner sent her to the author. Tests found her still allergic to all the items she was previously treated for. She was treated again for the first basic three items and she began feeling better. During the fourth treatment, while the treatment was in process, one of the toddlers from the waiting area wandered into the treatment room. The doctor stopped the treatment until the toddler was removed from the room. The patient inquired the reason for the pause while the child was in the room. When she was told that the presence of the third person could steal her treatment, she knew why she had not passed the previous 62 treatments.

Her two-year-old accompanied her to the practitioner's office and ran around in the room or clung to her feet during her visit. Her daughter was very sick with sinusitis, frequent bronchitis and colds when the mother had begun the treatments. After Mary received just a few NAET treatments, the child regained her health rather quickly. In this case, the daughter was being treated through Mary as a surrogate while Mary received no benefit without the practitioner or patient being aware of it.

Patients should learn MRT so they can test the allergy to the items before they buy at the market. One may have treated for all the Basics, yet all of a sudden, can react to eggs, milk, vegetable, fruits, etc. They may not be reacting to the original item here; it may be the pesticide or other chemicals in it. If the patient is able to test himself/herself, he/she can live with confidence. After clearing the Basics, and learning to test everything, the chances of getting sick from the allergens are very limited.

Special care may be needed if a patient has a specific problem, like alcoholism, gluten allergy, diabetes, milk allergy, smoking, drugs like penicillin, chemotherapy drugs, radiation, etc. Please check with your practitioner for information.

ALCOHOLISM

Patients with the h/o alcoholism, may need repeated treatments on B-complex vitamins, especially B12 and Paba. They will need mega doses of vitamin B-complex supplementation. Complete all the ten Basics, and yeast before treating the alcohol. They should be checked and treated for emotional components.

Cigarette smoke, drugs, cosmetics, drug addictions, caffeine addiction, etc. can be treated after the ten Basics.

CIGARETTE SMOKE

When one treats for cigarette smoking, inhalation of cigarette smoke while treating the spinal segment is necessary to get the complete treatment. How can you make the smoke sample? Take a 1/2 liter jar with a lid. Place some wet paper or cotton balls in the jar. Fill up the jar with exhaled cigarette smoke and close the lid tight until you are ready to be treated with NAET. While receiving NAET spinal treatment, the patient needs to inhale the smoke, then smell or smoke of cigarettes will not bother you at a future contact.

PERFUME

If someone is allergic to perfumes, spray few drops of different perfumes into a glass container with cotton balls at the bottom. Then treat the same way as you would treat cigarette smoke. Smell from flowers, new fabrics, chemicals, formaldehyde, building materials, paints, paint thinners, nail polish, molds, popcorn, coffee brewing, cooking smell, smell from deep fried oils, spices, herbs, hair products, newspaper, inks, etc. should be treated this way.

CONCRETE, CERAMICS, WOOD, AND BUILDING MATERIALS.

Many people react violently to ceramic cups, knife, knife-handle, mugs, tiles, marbles, concrete floors, driveways, wood furniture, wood work, paints, building materials, etc. Patients suffer from general body aches, joint pains, restlessness, weakness of the knees, ankles, or the whole limb while walking on the concrete or tiled surface and frequent falling down on the floors. Samples of the particular allergen should be collected and treated in such cases.

TREATING FOR ATMOSPHERIC CHANGES

HEAT

You can also test the patient for atmospheric changes. Many people have problems in extreme weather. Some people are very sensitive to heat. Some patients suffer from extreme fatigue and irritability during summer time. When the atmosphere begins to cool they feel better. Holding a couple of ounces of hot water in a glass jar can make the sample of heat. They need to avoid contact with any heat during the 25 hours after the treatment.

COLD

Some others are very sensitive to cold. Place an ice cube in a glass bottle to make a sample of cold. Then treat the patient while holding the bottle in his/her palm making contact with the fingers while receiving NAET. They need to avoid contact with cold during the 25 hours after the treatment.

HUMIDITY

Some people get sick in humid weather. They can get shortness of breath, asthma, swelling of the body, skin disorders, mental confusion, etc. To make sample of humidity: Take a 1/2 - litter jar with a narrow mouth and fill the jar half way with boiling water. Feel the steam at the finger tips while receiving NAET.

HIGH ALTITUDE

Some people get shortness of breath in high altitude. Oxygen content of the air falls very low in higher altitude. Carbon-dioxide is more predominant there. How do you treat for this problem? Fill up a paper or plastic bag with exhaled air and ask the patient to feel the air with the fingertips while giving NAET.

TREATING FOR CLOUDS

Many people complain of various levels of discomfort (migraines, asthma, shortness of breath, joint pains, depression, etc.), when there are lots of clouds in the sky, or before a heavy wind or a storm, . Oxygen content of the air falls very low during these episodes. Carbon-dioxide is more predominant there. How do you treat for this problem? Fill up a paper bag or plastic bag with exhaled air and ask the patient to feel the air with the fingertips while giving NAET.

LOW ALTITUDE

Some people react to low altitude, morning ocean breeze, cold fog, etc. Make a sample of cold mist by filling up a jar halfway with ice cubes and have the patient feel the cold vapor with the fingertips while treating with NAET. You may sprinkle few drops of water on the ice to create more cold vapor.

DAMPNESS

Allergy to dampness is one of the major causes of asthma among asthma sufferers. Some people complain of asthma or sinus blockages in the early morning or after waking up in the morning. Usually dampness is the cause. Dampness and cold, dampness and mold, dampness and fungus are some other variations of dampness one may need to check. Paper towel wetted with cold water (ice water) makes the sample for dampness.

DRYNESS/ DRY HEAT

Dryness can cause simple dryness of the nostrils, eyes, skin, skin disorders like eczema, psoriasis, acne, and itching of the skin. Some people also get asthma due to dryness. Heat up a piece of paper towel or cloth towel in a micro-wave oven for few seconds and feel the dry heat from the towel while you receive NAET.

DROUGHT

Walking in a windy area especially after taking a shower or bath, or sleeping under a fan can cause headaches, common cold, runny nose, sinus blockage, sore throat, etc. in some people. They are simply allergic to wind. To create wind: Turn the fan on and make the patient feel the air at the fingertips while receiving NAET.

AIR-CONDITIONING

First treat freon, ice, mold, and moving air (use a table fan). Then, combine different samples like freon and ice cubes, ice and fan, mold and fan, etc. Then combine all the above samples and turn on a table fan next to the patient to create an air-conditioned atmosphere. Have them hold ice cubes, other samples in their hand and feel the breeze from the fan with the fingertips while doing NAET.

You cannot create samples of heat and cold in a vial like other allergens. You have to feel actual heat or cold with the fingertips. So you have to have hot water and ice cubes available in the office to treat these items.

EXERCISE AND BODY MOVEMENTS

People can be allergic to exercise and movements like walking, jogging, running, playing tennis, dancing, sailing, rowing, driving in the car, etc. Different movements make sensitive people very sick. Allergy to these movements can be treated through NAET; you can enjoy all the activities you like without any unpleasant reactions. Please check with your NAET practitioner to test you and treat you for your activities if necessary.

INTESTINAL DISORDERS

In the cases of chronic irritable bowel syndrome, Crohn's disease, ulcerative colitis, gluten allergy, etc., first treat them with basic ten, then treat with starch, spices, fats, dried beans, alcohol, vitamin E, food colors, food additives, gluten, wheat, and other combinations. One combination should be done on one visit. Do not try to treat too many items in one treatment. That can make the patient's condition worse. One cup of rice broth before each meal can help with the intestinal pain and discomfort in these cases. Patients should be encouraged to save a sample of all the items ingested in a day and treat the combined food at the end of the day or next day. This should be repeated every other day for 20-30 days. Various food groups will be treated this way, since most people eat different food items on different days. Reactions to food combining will be eliminated by treating this way.

DIABETES

In treating diabetes, one should take special care. First treat them with basics, then add sugar and/or insulin to the basics as combinations. Then, treat liver, gall bladder, pancreas, parasites, glycogen, glucagon, and combinations with sugar. Frequent gall bladder cleansing once every two-three months is advised to prevent any stone formation. If there are any gall stones, they should be removed by natural means. You should be checked for parasite infestation, should seek appropriate treatment if needed. Gall bladder stones and chronic irritation of liver and gall bladder can lead to diabetes. Persica and Rhubarb formula 1X3 times a day after meals can help prevent gall stone formation.

DEPRESSION

Patients with depression suffer allergy or deficiency to brain nutrients. After completing the basic fifteen treatments, they should be checked for hormones, serotonin, phenylalanine, tyrosine, and glutamine. Treat them alone, then in combination if necessary. After allergy elimination, these items should be supplemented in mega doses for few months. Please check with your NAET practitioner for information.

YEAST/ CANDIDA

Many people suffer from yeast/ candida problems. They should be treated for Basic ten, yeast mix, alcohol, yeast and common combinations, yeast and heavy metals especially mercury, yeast and sugar, yeast and parasites, yeast and bacteria, yeast and daily nutritional supplements, and yeast and mixture of daily food (to eliminate the food combining reactions). After treating for yeast and candida, patient should be placed on good cleansing program for few weeks.

VIRUS / BACTERIA

Apart from treating for the specific virus (EBV for example), bacteria (steptococcus, E.Coli, for example), patient's saliva, urine, other body secretions, and own blood should be treated with NAET. In severe cases, it is advisable to get a sample of actual bacteria or the infecting organism and treat with NAET to receive faster results. Within a few hours of virus attack if you can treat the patient with his/her saliva, after-effect of virus attack will be greatly reduced.

AUTO-IMMUNE DISORDERS, BLOOD DISORDERS/ HIGH PLATELETS/ LOW WHITE BLOOD CELLS/ LEUKEMIA/ CANCER/ CHRONIC FATIGUE/ FIBROMYALGIA/ARTHRITIS

Treat with basic 30 items from NAET list. Then treat the food combinations like breakfast, lunch and dinner together for few times. then treat body secretions and blood. Sometimes, these body fluids may have to be treated few times at different intervals, like every week, month or so to get the best maximum benefit.

FUNGUS/ PARASITES

Many people suffer from fungus and parasite infestations. They need to be treated separately and then in combination with blood, candida, mold, sugar, mercury, virus, bacteria, etc. You should check them with all possible combinations to isolate the one that is causing your problem.

All new patients should be encouraged to get a copy of the book titled, "Living Pain free with Acupressure" by Devi S. Nambudripad, available at each of the practitioner's office or at the book store. A simple technique to balance the body is explained on page 58. All NAET patients should learn this technique. If you do not understand the technique just by reading, please ask your practitioner to explain it further. This technique is to be used once or twice a day by NAET patients to achieve and maintain balance in the body and reduce unpleasant symptoms following any NAET treatment. This book contains acupressure treatment points for over 280 health problems. Temporary symptom relief can be achieved by using these specially designed acupressure points. The book has 133 illustrations with acupressure points marked in colors for most commonly seen health emergencies. This unique and practical book will assist the patients in keeping their unpleasant symptoms under control while going through NAET treatments.

NAET Practitioners should hold patient education meetings at least once a month during which patients can be educated about NAET treatment programs. Friends and family should be encouraged to come for the meetings. Patients can have support group meetings every so often and the doctor can get involved with the group.

PREPARATION FOR TREATMENTS

It is recommended to shop in advance for the food and other items used during the 25-hour period after the treatment. Food, gloves, mask, distilled water, fabrics, etc., are the items one may need during the 25-hour period. Another reason to shop before the treatments is that many times the stores are filled with odors (including cooking odors) that can cause a reaction in sensitive patients, and cause the patient to lose the treatment.

Patient should be encouraged to prepare the appropriate foods before coming for the treatment. Patient also should eat some food within an hour of receiving NAET treatment. NAET treatment should not be taken on an empty stomach.

Distilled water should be used with the treatments of salt mix, mineral mix, calcium mix and chemicals. When the patient is not treating for anything, he/she should be encouraged to drink a lot of spring water or purified water. Drinking lots of water (6-8 glasses of water) helps the energy to move freely through the energy meridians. One should not drink distilled water continuously. It can deplete the essential minerals from the body.

BASIC TREATMENTS

"What are the basic treatments, and why should you treat them first?" "Can't I treat for my allergy to the cat first?" " Can't I treat my allergy to dust first?" "I don't react to any food. I only want to treat my allergy to the pesticides. Can't you treat that first?" Almost everyone asks these questions.

The basic treatments include treatment for the essential nutrients, vitamins, minerals, and those that are needed for the normal physical, physiological and emotional functions of the human body. These nutrients are necessary to maintain a good immune system. NAET is a non-invasive, gentle, energy manipulation treatment. If the immune system is good, the energy can be manipulated with the least effort on the energy system. When one does not have a good immune system, allergic reactions are intensified. When one tries to treat a severe allergy without improving the immune system, reactions can be very unpleasant and severe. Sometimes, a sudden shift of energy can cause light-headedness or fainting spells. With poor immune conditions, one's energy flow could be slow and it may take a number of treatments to clear one allergy. The basic treatments consist of the essential nutrients that boost up the immune system absorbed from the regular food we eat every day. When one is allergic to the food or the nutrients in the food, one cannot absorb or assimilate nutrients from the food. Nutrients are absolutely necessary for normal body functions, growth and development, to repair wear and tear in the body, fight infections and diseases, prevent invasion of foreign energies or bacteria and for proper maintenance of bodily functions. When one is allergic to eggs, milk, fruits, vegetables, or grains, etc., one is also allergic to the nutrients contained in them like proteins, calcium, vitamin C, sugar, B-complex, etc. that are needed for various body and enzymatic functions.

Proteins are the most essential factors in our body. Allergy to proteins (eggs) can make one more susceptible to frequent colds, flu-like symptoms, bronchitis, sinusitis, pneumonia, many other infections and asthma, skin problems, hair problems like poor growth, falling hair, premature gray, breathing problems, digestive disorders, muscle and joint pains, fatigue and weakness of the muscles, poor blood circulation, high cholesterol, high blood pressure, water retention in the tissues, mental or manic disorders, poor memory, poor concentration, headaches, sleep disorders, irritability, and hyperactivity, etc.

Allergy to each nutrient like calcium (milk), vitamin C, B-complex, etc., prevents normal body functions and causes damages to the body tissue (please refer to a vitamin book to understand the functions of vitamins in the human body).

When one gets treated for all the 30-40 essential basic groups of foods and environmental items, one will begin to assimilate the essential nutrients from the foods being eaten every day. This will build a strong immune system. Sudden occurrences of colds, flu's, pains, and various other health problems including allergic reactions will easily be prevented.

The basic treatments encompass: proteins, calcium, vitamin C, B-complex, sugars, iron, vitamin A, trace minerals, sodium chloride, corn, grains, artificial sweeteners, caffeine group, nuts, spices, fats, yeast group, vegetable proteins (beans), alcohol, gums, gelatin, starches, food colors, food additives, stomach acids, digestive enzymes, hormones, pesticides, parasites, chemicals, fabrics, and bacteria.

Allergies always affect the weakest tissue of a weak area in the body. If someone has a weak lung, the patients' allergies will affect the lung tissue. The patient will suffer from asthma, bronchitis or other respiratory disorders whenever they come in contact with an allergen. During elimination of most of the allergies, while the immune system improves, the presenting symptoms can change.

While being treated for many allergies, a woman with fibromyalgia noticed her general body ache had diminished. For months, any allergen she contacted caused her to have localized pain in her little finger. Her little finger pain was due to excessive toxins in the small bowel. It would be beneficial at this stage to eliminate the accumulated toxins with a few colonics or colon cleansers.

You do not have to be sick or bedridden to have NAET treatments. NAET can be used as a preventive health measure. Clearing the basic allergies helps to lead a normal life. For example: assume you have a minor sensitive-skin disorder. By clearing all the basic allergies your skin will improve. Then one day, you drink a glass of orange juice, and develop rashes and hives all over your body. Immediately, you would know that some foreign substance in the juice caused the rashes. You can take a few drops of the juice and self-treat with NAET. The rashes will disappear in a few minutes and you won't have to go to an emergency room for treatment of hives. If you have never been treated for the basic allergies and severe skin rashes appeared, you would not know which part of the food caused the rashes. You might have to go to the emergency room to get some relief. Thus, when one clears all the basic allergies, life becomes a lot easier. That is why I stress the importance of the basic treatments. If possible, every one (sick or not) should be treated for at least the basic ten. Better health can only be achieved through proper nutrients, and "proper nutrients" means non-allergic nutrients. Better health through right nutrients can give you a higher quality of life for longer time.

ORDER OF TREATMENTS

It is very important to follow the order of treatments as given in the following pages. The items are listed according to priority of importance to the body.

The First item to treat in the NAET program is the Egg mix (protein), because the human body depends on protein for its normal every day function. Egg protein is close to a complete protein that our bodies recognize. Even if we do not eat eggs, our body recognizes the egg protein, due to the similarities to the human body proteins.

The Second preferred item is Calcium, the next important item for body function. Calcium is necessary for any movement in the body, walking, running, eating, heart beating etc. These require a certain amount of calcium in the blood. If the patients are allergic to calcium, they cannot absorb calcium from their food to run daily, normal body functions. The result may be fatigue, body aches, muscle aches, constipation, (the colon is unable to relax), hyperactivity, irritability, high blood pressure, inability to calm down and relax, or insomnia, etc.

The Third important item is vitamin C, needed for the growth, development, repairing wear and tear of the cells and tissues, clearing poisons from the blood etc. Vitamin C is a very good antioxidant. After the vitamin C treatment, most fruits and vegetables eaten will be non-reactive. The patients can begin to add more healthy foods into their diet list after treating for vitamin C. Many environmental substances contain Vitamin C, such as grasses, pollen, soaps and detergents with citric acid (lemon scented), strawberry or mint flavored tooth past, mouthwash, etc. After the Basic treatments, reactions to environments will be reduced. Vitamin C allergy causes repeated bladder infections, frequent yeast and other infections, poor circulation, skin conditions and digestion, etc.

The Fourth item is B-Complex. B-complex vitamins are necessary for various functions such as enzymatic and nerve functions. In addition to treating the B-complex as a group, it may be necessary, to treat the individual B vitamins separately. Check each B to see whether it should be treated individually. B vitamins are the food for the nerves. With a starving nervous system we cannot do any work in the body. Sensitivities can occur when our nervous system does not function normally. A good, efficient nervous system is necessary for clear thinking and other brain functions. Allergy to B-complex vitamins and malabsorption cause various brain disorders like hyperactivity, attention deficit disorders, autism, restlessness, sleep disorders, depression, addictions to drugs, alcohol, smoking, overeating, skin disorders, body ache, fatigue, etc.

The Fifth item is Sugar. Sugar is very necessary for the normal absorption and assimilation of B-complex vitamins. B-complex vitamins travel in the body from one place to another with the help of sugar molecules. Sugar works as the seeing-eye-dog for the B-complex vitamins. If allergic to B-complex, one can suffer from malfunctioning of the nervous system. If allergic to sugar, the same thing can happen, because B-complex cannot function without sugar. Various nervous disorders, addictions, overeating, sinusitis, susceptibility to frequent infections, alcoholism, smoking, insomnia, fatigue, allergies, hyperactivity, hypersensitivity etc. could be due to allergy to B-complex, sugar or both. After these five major treatments, patients should be encouraged to eat food from these five groups right away, so they can begin to feel better. Most people begin to see dramatic health changes when they complete the first five treatments.

Iron, vitamin A, mineral mix, salt mix, corn mix and grain mix are the next five items in the basic-ten series. These ten items are important in building-up and maintaining a good immune system. If the patient has a strong immune system, the patient could get through the NAET treatments easier. When one has a weak immune system, she or he may experience some side effects like light-headedness, nausea, lack of energy, etc., while going through the 25-hour period after the treatment. Experience has shown us that one may get through NAET, with just one treatment per item, if the exact order of treatment is followed.

On occasion, we have seen, someone hurry into doing Corn Mix, Grain Mix or Formaldehyde without completing the first ten items. This patient may take many treatments (anywhere from two to fifteen) on that item, before they can get through the treatment or feel comfortable. In some cases, someone with a strong immune system may be able to get through the treatment, without side effects to any item, even if treated out of order. The doctor should be able to detect who needs to follow the order strictly, through MRT testing. It is all right to treat out of order once testing detects the patient has a good immune system.

Generally, it is advised to complete ten basic treatments before beginning treatments for environmental and other items such as: chemicals, fabrics, pollens, weeds, grasses, insects, hormones, thyroid, medications, radiation, chemotherapy drugs, formaldehydes, paints, perfumes, animals etc.

If one follows the order as given in the list of basic allergens, it is possible that the patient will take less number of treatments, since one overlaps another. For example: when treated for vitamin A, most people do not react to beta-carotene, carrots, fish or shellfish mix. If one decides to treat fish mix as a first item, they will consequently have to treat fish mix, shellfish mix, vitamin A and beta-carotene separately.

TREATING FOOD ALLERGY FIRST

People with environmental allergy will also have food allergy. Most of the environmental allergens contain food elements. Grass, weeds, etc. contain vitamin C, vitamin A, minerals, vitamin B, etc. In most cases, when treated for nutrients, their environmental reactions will reduce greatly. It is easy to stay away from grasses, trees and weeds etc., but it is not easy to stay away from food for too long. When treated for nutrients, one can begin to eat nutritious foods and able to absorb nutrients from that food. This will help strengthen the immune system and the patient can go through the treatments easier.

FREQUENCY OF THE TREATMENTS

NAET requires that a patient stay completely away from the offending allergen for a period of 25 hours after a treatment. This involves careful restriction of the diet during the treatment period for food allergies and regulation of the environment as well. Due to this reason, we recommend that you preferably undergo one treatment per week if you are very sick, or your immune system has been lowered, caused by allergies or long term illnesses. If you are fairly healthy, yet have many allergies, you may be able to take two treatments per week. You may leave that decision to your practitioner if you wish to speed up your treatment sessions. Whatever the case, the allergen being treated should be completely desensitized before treating a new allergen.

If one allergen is not completely desensitized, the patient can get exacerbation of existing complaints. For example: treating for sugars, the presenting symptoms are skin irritations, eczema, psoriasis, acne etc. If the treatment for sugar is incomplete, the skin condition can get worse. If, by MRT, the practitioner is unable to detect any weakness on the treating allergen at that time, please do not treat another allergen. Instead, wait two days to a week, then repeat the test for that allergen, and with all combinations. The patient should be feeling better by then if the treatment is completed. If the patient is still reactive to the allergen, the practitioner will be able to find it at this time. After a few days' rest, the body will reveal the weakness towards the allergen.

Let's look at this situation. The practitioner could not find any weakness for the particular allergen after testing the patient 25 hours following the initial treatment. Yet, the patient was not feeling well, or was feeling worse. One of the following could be the cause:

1. The practitioner could be suffering from an allergic reaction. His/her blockage is not allowing the detection of the patient's allergy.

2. The energy of the practitioner or the patient is reversed or switched.

3. The practitioner or the patient is dehydrated or starving for food.

4. The practitioner is not very skilled at MRT.

5. Patient is overpowering the practitioner.

6. Patient is too weak and the practitioner is overpowering the patient.

7. Patient has passed about 90 % of the treatment, and the last 10% is too difficult to detect immediately after 25 hours.

8. Patient has passed the physical and chemical levels. The emotional level needs to be treated again.

9. If the patient is getting treated for a large group (like vitamin B or C, etc.), one or some of the items are not completed.

10. The patient was not cleared for individual items in the combination treatment before she was treated for mixed energies. For example: before clearing the basic ten, the practitioner decided to treat an acute reaction to a chocolate chip cookie, because the patient reacted to the cookie on that day and has no time to treat for the basic ten. In such a case, the practitioner should check the patient for the allergy to the individual items in the cookie, i.e.: flour, sugar, chocolate chip, salt, egg, fat, additives, colors, water, the baking pan, etc. Then do a temporary clearance on each item before he/she performs NAET for the actual cookie. At a later point, when the patient feels better, treat her for all the Basic allergens.

11. Patient did not wait for the specified restricted time (usually 25 hours, or as it is detected by the practitioner) before she came in contact with the allergen. If the patient comes in contact with the treated allergen before completing the 25 hours, do not panic. He/she should wash her hands immediately or rub the palms together for few seconds and give herself a balancing treatment (Page 58 in the "Living Pain-Free" book by this author). The practitioner and patient should work together to solve the problem, if such a need arises.

When a patient fails a treatment, and for some reason decides to stop the NAET treatments, please do not panic. NAET is not a dangerous technique. It does not cause any severe or permanent damage on anyone or any system. It is a mild, gentle, non-invasive, precise, energy manipulation technique.

If the practitioner is successful in removing the energy blockage and establishing the energy flow in the right direction, the result will be great and the patient will get the expected results. If the energy flow did not get established in the right direction during the attempt, the patient is not adding more blockages to the existing energy blockages. They will still have their blockages as before. The attempt to remove the blockages will make them tired or uncomfortable for a short period. For the first couple of days they may not feel very good. If this happens they are to drink 8-10 glasses of non-allergic water a day. The reaction will wear off gradually. In a week or two, they will reach their pre-NAET condition.

The body is very good in adapting and adjusting to any environment. The body will adapt to its normal self as it has adjusted to all the allergies throughout their lives before they began NAET. But it is very important to drink lots of water. Water enhances the energy flow through the energy pathways.

Some allergens can be contacted in unlikely places. This guide has been prepared to alert unsuspecting patients to some common hideouts for these offending substances. Some of the restrictions for particular items during the 25-hour period may seem inconvenient. We suggest preparation according to the guidelines outlined in this book to simplify and speed up the process and avoid any unintentional contact with the allergen for which the patient is being treated.

25 HOUR RESTRICTION

There are 12 major energy pathways (meridians) in the body. Energy molecules take 2 hours to pass through one meridian when one has normal energy flow. During the NAET treatment, the normal energy flow of that particular molecule of that allergen is established through the energy pathways. If the energy molecule can complete its travel without interruption and return to the original starting point in 24-25 hours, the uninterrupted journey of that particular energy is imprinted in the brain as harmless or beneficial energy. The brain will be friendlier towards that energy or item in any future contact with that substance.

Occasionally, the patient may overcome allergy to the treated item in a few minutes, or in a few hours. In the majority of cases it takes 25 hours to clear. In many instances, the patient may still experience severe symptoms even in the case of a minor blockage, until the blockage is cleared with NAET. The practitioner can also find the approximate time needed for clearance through MRT testing.

Rarely, in some cases it may take 30-40 hours to clear the allergy depending on the severity. If one finds out that he/she falls in the group who takes 30 hours or more to clear, they should take extra caution for more than 30 hours each time whenever treated. We suggest that you adhere to the avoidance for at least 25 hours all the time. If one cleared in 2 hours or ten hours and still followed the 25 hours restriction, there is nothing to lose. If one fails the treatment due to negligence (not avoiding the allergen for a good 25 hours or whatever time is needed), he/she may have to go through the treatment again. That means, making another trip to the doctor, spending more money and another depressing day of avoiding the allergen!

Less allergic or sensitive patients have been known to clear the allergy sooner than 25 hours following treatment. They may be able to touch the item without losing the treatment. If you are a highly allergic patient you should avoid any contact with the allergen during the required time.

Cleansing and flushing of the allergic foods and nutrients from the system takes place after the treatments. This continues for the next 24 to 25 hours following the NAET treatment. I strongly recommend avoiding the allergic group for at least 25 hours following the treatment to achieve the added benefit of cleansing the years' old poison from one's system. Patients who do not observe 25-hour clearance for an allergen, tend to come up with many combination treatments per item in the future. If the patient takes good care for 25 hours, they take fewer combinations on the same allergen and less future treatments on other items.

After the 25 hours, the doctor rechecks the patient's response to the allergen with MRT. If the MRT is strong, the patient should use a small amount of the allergen and test the physical response to the allergen. If there is any further adverse reaction, report to the doctor immediately and if necessary repeated treatments on the substance or in combination with other items, should be given.

ANAPHYLAXIS

If someone is severely allergic to the allergen (with the h/o anaphylactic shock, etc.), special care should be taken during the treatment. Patient can be tested and treated through a surrogate for the best results. During the treatment, patient should not hold the sample for usual 15-20 minutes. After passing the treatment, the patient may still be afraid to eat or use the allergen. Please advise the patient to hold the item in his/her palm for a few minutes to an hour to see if there are any adverse reactions in the body. The patient can continue to hold the allergen every day for a few minutes (three-four days consecutively). At the end of the test period, if the outcome is satisfactory, he/ she can try to eat or use it. This method is very useful in testing the effectiveness of NAET in patients with extreme reactions to drugs, penicillin, milk, eggs, shell fish, peanuts, peanut butter, or latex products etc., before reintroducing the substances.

EAT OR FAST

One of the frequently asked questions is "Must I eat during the 25 hours or can I fast?" NAET treatment may appear to be an easy treatment. But various energy changes and energy rearrangements along the energy meridians are taking place during and after the treatments. Energy rearrangement takes a lot of energy. One can replenish the needed energy from food intake. So, fasting is not recommended after NAET treatments. Eat the minimum number of foods from the recommended list of items. Please avoid too many variations of foods soon after the treatments. Limit the food intake to this limited variety of items. Eat any amount from one or two categories. Different foods or food groups take different levels of energy for digestion. When one eats too many varieties following the treatments, the brain may need to spend more energy digesting the various items. Eating one or two items helps the cleansing process.

The lists of food that can be eaten safely are given in this book after each allergen (in the next few pages). We have given just a few items after each treatment. One may find more items to eat safely after each category of allergen. But please limit the items for your own benefit.

After completion of Basic Ten, the patient is advised to collect his/her breakfast items together, lunch items together and dinner items together, and bring them to the office for treatment. This food combining treatment will continue for a couple of weeks. This will reduce the need for combination treatments.

When treating for the environmental items like grass, dust, trees etc., the patient is instructed to bring samples from his/her neighborhood to the office. Collecting samples of local pollen or dust: Leave a flat dish with water for couple of days in an open area near your house when the wind blows. After the wind settles down, pour the water into a glass bottle and take it to your doctor to treat. This can be treated along with the sample in the doctor's treatment kit. This rule can be applied to vegetable mix, household chemicals, vitamin supplements, etc.

Please do not treat children, extremely weak patients, elderly patients, and debilitated patients with more than one item at a time. Plenty of clean, non-allergic water (6-8 glasses /day) should be taken throughout the day. Herbal teas can be taken with all treatments except with vitamin C, B-complex, and spices. Salt can be used with all treatments except for salt treatment.

EATING REFINED FOOD

Refined foods should be avoided as much as possible. Eat more allergy-free complex carbohydrates and fresh fruits and vegetables. In the initial stage, cook well if it is hard to digest. If you are non-vegetarian, eat non-allergic lean meats. Avoid excess fat consumption. Excess fat in the food will slow down the energy circulation through the energy meridians. White rice should be used with B complex, iron, sugar and vitamin E treatments. Brown rice can be used with all other treatments.

HOW ABOUT A JUICE FAST?

Fasting with juices is highly recommended after clearing the Vitamin C group. Extremely weak, tired, chronically sick patients, patients with malabsorption problems, immune deficient patients, patients with cancer, Aids, Chronic Fatigue Syndromes, gastric ulcers, fever, etc. should be drinking lots of juices initially. Juices do not require much energy for digestion. Nutrients from the juices can be assimilated easily. After the patients gain enough strength, they can begin to eat nutritious solid foods and increase roughage. Vegetable juices should be taken more. Fruit juices should be limited to one or two glasses daily. When on a juice diet, he/she should, in addition, drink 6-8 glasses of non-allergic clean water. Water will help the assimilation of nutrients.

FOOD CRAVING DURING TREATMENT

Most of the time, when one is treated for an allergen with NAET, she/he may experience an unusual craving for that particular item. For example, if some one is treated for salt, sugar, or spices, she/he may crave salt, sugar (ice cream), or spicy food respectively during the 25-hour period. Some people may experience withdrawal symptoms. If they resist the temptation and follow the restriction for the 25-hour period, the craving will subside the next day. That allergen will probably never bother them again, during the rest of their lives unless the items are chemically contaminated.

Soon after a successful completion of treatment, one may crave the particular food for a few days. For example, after finishing treatment for B- complex vitamins, one may crave bread and grain products. This is because the long-term allergy has created a huge deficiency of the essential nutrients in his/her body. The brain simply demands to bring more of the essential nutrients into the body. In such cases the patient may need to take large doses of vitamin or mineral supplements for a certain period. In cases of pain disorders, one may need to take large amount of calcium, magnesium, zinc, phosphorus, etc., for few weeks. The doctor will help to decide the duration and amount of large doses of vitamin/mineral supplementation.

NEED FOR SUPPLEMENTS

After completing the treatment for the essential nutrients (like Calcium, B Complex, Vitamin A, Iron, Vitamin E, trace minerals, mineral supplements and Amino Acids) it may be advisable to take supplements for a few months to reduce the deficiency, to assist the body to recover faster.

People who take appropriate supplements after treatments usually get better faster than people who depend on only food to supplement their needs. One should be careful to check the allergy to the particular vitamin/supplements before taking them. Even though the patient was treated for vitamins like B Vitamins, C Vitamins, Minerals, Enzymes, etc. they react with various, unusual health problems just by taking allergic products. So each container should be checked for allergy before taking it. Another concern about supplements is the possibility of overdose. After NAET treatments, the body is able to assimilate 80-100% of the nutrients from the products consumed. Check the daily need frequently and adjust the dosage accordingly. Overdose can produce allergy-like symptoms. Overdose can be treated with NAET as an allergy. In case of overdose, hold the item that is overdosed and repeat the NAET every 10 minutes until the patient feels better.

NAET METHOD TO EVALUATE THE NEED FOR SUPPLEMENTS

This method can be used to determine the adequate dosage of prescription medication, vitamin-mineral supplements, herbal supplements, laxatives, amount of caloric intake, etc.

Find an indicator muscle (Find any strong muscle. Please read "Say Goodbye to Illness," chapter 6 for more information on muscle response testing.)

Have the patient hold one vitamin pill (e.g. B-Complex, calcium) in his free hand.
Test the indicator muscle.

If weak, then the patient is allergic to the pill. Treat the patient for that pill using NAET, or they can go to any NAET practitioner who can eliminate their allergies by using NAET.

If his/her indicator muscle is strong in the presence of one pill, add more pills one by one into the patient's hand, until the indicator muscle goes weak. When the arm muscle goes weak, stop adding pills to the hand.

Now count the pills in the hand. The total number in the hand is the total deficiency on that day in the present condition.

This number can be anywhere from 1-2 pills to many thousands depending on the deficiency. For example: in certain nerve disorders, the total amount of Vitamin B-complex deficiency can be as high as 20-30 thousand grams.

If the deficiency is 1-6 pills, one may not need to take supplements. Regular balanced meals will provide the requirements.

If the deficiency is more than 6-10 pills (or the amount equals 6-10 times recommended daily dosage (RDA), then one should supplement one pill daily. If the deficiency is calculated in many tens, hundreds, or thousands, supplement the person with 4-6 times the recommended daily dosage of that particular supplement, until the deficiency is taken care of. Never supplement more than 4-6 times the RDA amount on any given day. In case of a huge deficiency, when someone is taking mega-doses of supplements (4-6 times the RDA amount), then, the supplements should be checked every three days. If one continues to take the supplements in mega-doses after displacing the deficiency, they can easily overdose on the supplements. They may experience allergy-like or other unusual symptoms when they overdose on supplements.

When that person is no longer deficient, he/she can eat a balanced meal or take a multivitamin-mineral supplement. When a patient is no longer allergic to a substance, the body will naturally demonstrate a need for that item. This helps to bring the body to a balance by supplementing the long-term deficiency caused by the allergy. It is essential to supplement appropriately to achieve better and faster results when the allergy is successfully treated. But one has to be careful not to overdose with vitamins or drugs. After the NAET treatments, body will absorb vitamins easily. So daily requirements can decrease even with taking a small dosage of vitamin. If one takes too much it can become toxic. Use the same technique to measure the toxicity.

Supplements in mega doses are often needed for a number of months in the following cases: arthritis, fibromyalgia, chronic fatigue, any chronic problems related to allergy, hair loss, constipation, degenerative diseases, cancer, etc.

COMBINATION TREATMENTS

The stomach has strong acids to help break down the food we eat. The intestinal tract produces strong alkaline juices. When the food mixes with the acid, a chemical reaction occurs. The end result of any chemical reaction is a new product and heat. The new product produces new characteristics and thus new energy. One may be allergic to this new product's energy. This reaction can be reproduced by combining the energy of the food and acid. If there is an incompatibility between this new energy and the patients', it can be demonstrated by muscle testing. If there is a reaction, it can be eliminated the same way as the individual allergen.

Likewise, in advance, we can find the reaction between an allergen and alkalinity and RNA/DNA. Heat is being produced in the body during any chemical process. Sometimes, proper digestive steps do not take place when ice (cold) is consumed. It is necessary to clear the reaction between heat and the food, or cold and the food. In the same way an allergen can react with the organs, i.e.: allergen and lung, allergen and heart, allergen and brain etc. Sometimes an allergen can react with female hormones, male hormones, pituitary gland secretion, adrenaline, serotonin, pineal gland, one's blood, sweat, etc.

In cases where an allergy is inherited from parents and grand parents, one may need many combination treatments to overcome the allergic reactions completely. The possible combinations are allergen and stomach acids; allergen and alkalinity of the intestinal juices (Base); allergen and RNA, DNA; allergen and heat (salt and heat for example); allergen and cold (freon and cold in case of an allergy to air-conditioning); Individual vital organs (stomach, heart, lung, liver, gall bladder, pancreas, small intestine, etc.); allergen and liver as in pesticides and liver; allergen and pancreas (sugar and pancreas in cases of diabetes); allergen and kidney (salted nuts and kidney); allergen and lungs (bacteria and lung in case of lung infection, bronchitis, etc.); Allergen and stomach (garlic bread and stomach tissue in a case with acidity of the stomach after eating garlic bread); allergen and urinary bladder (cotton underpants with urinary bladder tissue in a patient with frequent bladder infection where one is allergic to cotton underpants); allergen and colon (gluten and colon); allergen and gall bladder (gall bladder and oils); allergen and heart (sulfites and heart); allergen and brain enzymes (serotonin and brain tissue); allergen and hormones; allergen and emotion; allergen and sugar; allergen and eczema; hormones and calcium (Osteoporosis); hormones and sugar (hot flashes); hormones and salt (P.M.S.); hormones, sugar and heat (hot flashes); sugar and spleen (sugar craving, fatigue); sugar and liver (liver headaches); sugar and brain tissue (brain fog, brain fatigue); fats and brain tissue (sensation of heaviness in the brain); fats, sugar and blood vessels (high serum triglycerides); calcium, fats and blood vessels (arteriosclerosis); bacteria and lung tissue (pneumonia); proteins and lymph (edema or water retention in the tissues); amino acid and stomach acids (hyperactivity, autism); amino acid and digestive enzymes (abdominal bloating); fats, cold and hormones (obesity); fats and vitamin C (obesity); vitamin C and blood vessels (bruising easily, Raynaud's disease); cholesterol and blood (high serum cholesterol); calcium and sugar and proteins (scleroderma); etc.

After completing the first 30 groups, it is advisable to collect all the breakfast items together, lunch items together, dinner items together and treat each group separately first, then combine breakfast, lunch and dinner together to remove the reaction seen due to food combining. Many people react by abdominal bloating, poor absorption, etc., when they eat carbohydrate and protein together; yogurt and meat, proteins and fats, etc. NAET treatments on combined multiple foods can easily remove that problem. The patient will be able to eat carbohydrate, proteins, fats and spices all at once and absorb the nutrients from the group without any unpleasant reaction.

EMOTIONAL ALLERGY

Many times, origin of the physical symptoms could be traced back to some unresolved emotional trauma. A woman in her fifties complained of hypoglycemia since childhood. She was found to be very allergic to sugar. When she was treated for sugar with NAET, she cleared her physical and chemical allergy. But emotional allergy remained the same and her hypoglycemic reaction was exaggerated. On further investigation she recalled, at five years of age, being restricted from eating sugar. Her parents told her sugar was bad for her health. One day, as a gesture of love, a family friend gave her a box full of chocolate bars. But as soon as the friend left the house, her mother snatched the box from her and flushed the chocolates in the toilet before she had a chance to eat one. The child felt very bad and cried for a long time. Her mother did not take time to explain the reason for her insensitive behavior. This puzzled the child and left an unhealed wound in her heart and brain. Ever since that event, for 48 years, with each contact with sugar or sugar products, she experienced unpleasant reactions, misdiagnosed as hypoglycemia. When she was treated for this emotional blockage with NAET, she no longer suffered from hypoglycemia.

A young man of 32, was tested allergic to almost all food items. After treating for the Basics, he still got sick and complained of nausea after each meal. He tried to eat just few items that was absolutely cleared for allergies by NAET and confirmed by MRT. He was tested for emotional blockage by MRT and found he was fearful to eat any food that was tied in with his childhood. As he was growing up, his abusive and maniac father abused his mother verbally and physically and often beat her or threw the dishes at her while eating. Watching all this horrible incidents, frightened young Jim often lost his appetite and went without eating. This unfortunate incidents left deep wounds in his mind in association with foods. When he was treated for this fear of childhood, he was able to eat food without getting sick.

Suppose two people were fighting while eating popcorn. One got upset and walked out of the room. The second person was very angry with the person who left the room. He was thinking of a way to solve the problem or to get back at him, and kept eating the popcorn without paying any attention to his eating. In fact, at a later point he may not even remember that he ate all of that popcorn. While he was eating popcorn his brain was stimulated with anger and resentment. That was forgotten. However, the brain was aware of eating popcorn, and it was forced to associate this with anger and resentment. The brain, always watching over our welfare, makes a note of this association. In a future contact with popcorn, the brain will caution him about the previous episode of anger and resentment while he eats popcorn. This can mimic an allergic reaction.

After the successful completion of treatment for an allergen, the physical and nutritional allergy may never return. But the emotional allergy can return any number of times if one is not careful to avoid unpleasant things while eating or cooking. **It is very important to respect food preparation and consumption for better assimilation of the nutrients and thus one can avoid the recurrence of emotional allergies.**

DEVELOP GOOD EATING HABITS AND PREVENT EMOTIONAL BLOCKAGES

Avoid eating when under stress. Always have pleasant thoughts while eating and enjoy your food. You can play your favorite music while you eat whether you are eating alone or with your eating partner. When you send the food into your stomach accompanied with feelings of love and happiness, your body and mind will cherish the nutrients with love and happiness and help the body and mind to grow healthy.

Many people bless the food before they eat. This ritual gives a chance to clear the mind of all troubled emotions. Fill the mind with a sense of spirituality before eating, thus avoiding troubled emotions and food associations. Try to eat with people who share pleasant thoughts and make eating a pleasing event. Avoid fights, exchanging unpleasant words, bad news etc., while eating. This will prevent repeated emotional blockages associated with food.

DIET

NAET patients are encouraged to eat non-allergic food whenever possible. After three or four treatments, he/she is encouraged to eat strictly non-allergic foods from the groups that have already been treated. After completion of each treatment, add that group or item into his/her diet. This will help the patient to get through the rest of the treatments better and faster with limited unexpected reactions. NAET patients should drink 5-8 glasses a day of clear, non-allergic water.

EXERCISE

Regular exercise is very important to distribute the nutrients evenly in the body. Begin very slowly if one is very sick or out of practice with exercise. Ten minutes of any kind of exercise, twice a day is advisable. If someone feels joint pains or excessively tired after the exercise, it is advisable to take 500 milligrams of calcium before the exercise. Drink a large glass of water after the exercise to help eliminate the toxins produced during the exercise.

MASSAGE

Massages should be taken before the NAET treatment. Therapeutic massages improve circulation and thus help distribute nutrients. Massages help to rid the toxins produced during the treatments. The patient should drink a full glass of water after the massage to help eliminate the impurities produced. Vigorous exercise, massage, swimming, Jacuzzi, extreme hot baths etc., are not advisable after the NAET treatment. Wait at least 6 hours before engaging in any of these activities.

ACUPUNCTURE

Acupuncture is used to balance the body. Traditional acupuncture with many needles, etc., should be given to the patient before NAET. Other kinds of acupuncture treatments are not advisable during the 25 hours after the treatment. Just four, six or eight needles should be used on the balancing points to maintain homeostasis of the body after NAET. Balancing points always remain the same for most people. During the NAET treatment, many patients react differently to the needles. Some people feel pain and discomfort in varying degrees at the needle site, depending on the severity of the allergens. Severe reactions can be expected for the severe allergen. Reactions can be as follows: shooting pain, shock like pain, cramps, pulling like pain, dull and distended pain, red welts, etc., can be found around the needles. Most often they will disappear a few minutes after the needle insertion. If the redness continues beyond 15 minutes, it is advisable to retain the needle for a longer period of time. If the patient feels light headed, or experiences extreme emotional variations like agitation, anger, crying spells, etc., shortly after the stage-1 treatment (spinal treatment) or during the 20 minutes waiting period, the needles should be removed immediately (if they are on needles). Emotional blockages should be checked and treated right away. If the patient is alone or with others in the waiting area and experiences such unusual symptoms, she/he should notify the practitioner right away.

After 20 minutes of treatment, if a drop of blood appears when the needle is removed, it is a good response to the treatment. Toxic energy will have a chance to come out of the body through the bloodlet area. If there is a red streak, welt or redness around the needle, the needle should be left in for a few more minutes until the reaction diminishes. If there is edema, a black and blue mark, etc., present at the needle site after removing the needle, it denotes that the allergen being treated is a strong one.

Sometimes, the patient can experience various types of energy movements, at various parts of the body, while the patient is holding the allergen during the 20 minutes after the stage-1 treatment. If the sensation is too uncomfortable, the patient should not hold the allergen. You can move the allergen from the palm and place it next to the body.

If the patient reports that he/she tends to get severe allergic reactions to an allergen (h/o anaphylaxis) please treat her/him through a surrogate. If someone reacts violently to the allergen, it is not necessary to hold the item in the hand during the stage-2 treatment (needle, acupoint massage, 20 minutes waiting period, etc.). If the patient had a huge bruise, swelling etc. at the site of the needle, if it caused tissue damage in the surrounding area, the doctor should avoid inserting needles at that particular acupuncture point for approximately a week. If there is a hematoma, pain in the needle area, please apply hot moist compresses for a few minutes, it will be resolved shortly. In a day or so the tissue will go back to normal.

CONSIDERATIONS FOR UNUSUAL CONDITIONS

NAET treatment should be avoided in the first three days' of menstrual cycle. Acupuncture is not advised during the first three days of menstruation and in pregnant women.

Young children under 15, extremely weak patients, pregnant women, women who are in their first three days of menstrual cycle, patients who are afraid of acupuncture needles, patients with history of acupuncture needle shocks, patient with skin infections, swelling of the limbs, etc., should not be needled. Massages on the acupoints will be sufficient to complete the treatment.

Patients with spinal deformity, severe case of spinal segmental degeneration, moderate to severe scoliosis, severe arthritis, patients with highly sensitive back, recent back surgery, abnormal growths on the spine or on the back, young children under two, etc., should not be treated directly on the back. Use a surrogate in such cases.

RECORD KEEPING

Space is provided in this guidebook for the patient to keep a record of individual treatments and notes of progress.

In addition, pages are provided to help the patient start a food diary and chart exposure to other potential allergens and the appearance of any symptoms. After clearing for the major allergens, one might notice numerous reactions to various simple items. When one's body gets rid of severe allergies, other allergies could easily be noticed. By maintaining a diary, the patient is able to help the doctor pick up the next most important item to be treated. These records of the frequency of reaction to certain products along with dates, may prove helpful in uncovering unrecognized allergens.

A patient reacted to anything she ate from her freezer. More investigation proved that she was allergic to the fungus and molds found in the freezer. Another patient's complaints of frequent angina pain, sinus problems, arrhythmia, frequent eye inflammation, etc. were completely relieved after treating for fungus. Even though she was not eating frozen foods, every day she would pet her dog who was suffering from some unknown skin problem related to fungus. In this case, the dog was also treated for fungus, and the dog's skin problem improved.

One patient had a reaction to elm trees since childhood. Since she was not getting better with food treatment, she was treated for elm trees. Her condition worsened with the initial treatment, breaking out in huge hives all over her body. She needed repeated treatments for elm tree for one week. At the end of the week, not only did her skin clear up, most of her other allergies improved.

This guidebook is intended to help patients understand the importance of avoiding contact with the allergen for which they are being treated during the 25 hour period, and to make that process easier for them. In no way do these guidelines replace the advice of the professional carrying out the treatments, and all patients are encouraged to discuss any individual problems thoroughly with their doctor.

CLINIC RULES

Rules may vary from one NAET office to another. However, the following are typical of what you should expect in any office or clinic carrying out these treatments:

1. Please do not wear any perfume, perfumed powder, strong smelling deodorant, hair spray, or after shave when you come in to the clinic for treatments.

2. There is no smoking allowed in (or around) the office. Please do not wear clothes that smell like smoke or paint. Other patients could react to these smells.

3. Please wash your hands before and after the treatment. After the treatment, if the patient cannot wash his/her hands, vigorous rubbing of the hands for 30 seconds will be sufficient.

4. Do not exercise for 6 hours after the treatment.

5. Avoid exposure to extreme hot or cold temperature after the treatment.

6. Please take a shower before you come for a treatment.

7. Do not bathe or shower until 6 hours after the treatment.

8. Do not eat or chew gum or candy during treatment.

9. Do not cross your hands or feet in the time (about 20 minutes) between treatment and recheck.

10. Do not read or touch other objects during the 20 minutes following the stage-1 treatment because contact with other substances during this period could cause your treatment to fail.

11. Wear no or minimum jewelry when you come for a treatment.

12. Remember to check with your doctor for the item you treated, after 25 hours, and at least within one week (to make sure you have completed the treatment. If you did not complete the treatment, your existing symptoms may continue for a long time).

13. To insure maximum progress with your treatments maintain your own treatment and food diary.

14. You may need to wear gloves while you get treated for environmental substances like mineral mix, metals, water, leather, formaldehyde, fabric, wood, mold, etc. You may need to wear a mask while you get treated for chemical smells, pollens, dust and dust mites, perfumes, etc.

15. Always eat before you come for the treatment. You should not take NAET treatments and acupuncture when you are hungry.

16. Do not eat heavy meals after acupuncture.

17. Drink lots of water after NAET and acupuncture treatments to help cleanse the toxins produced during the treatment.

18. Please do not stop any other treatment you are on - like any medication, therapy, chiropractic treatments, massages etc. It is good for your body to have a general body massage immediately before the NAET or 6 hours after the NAET treatments. Massages can help to improve the energy flow through the energy pathways. If you are taking lots of vitamins and herbs, or any particular drug, you may continue them as before if you think that they are helping you. But when you get treated for the food containing a particular vitamin, herb, or substance, you may be asked to stop using that for 25 hours following that particular treatment.

19. NAET treatment will not interfere with any other treatment. In fact, if you can keep your presenting symptoms under control with whatever method you are using, NAET treatment will be a lot easier.

PATIENT'S CHART OF MAJOR SYMPTOMS

Before Treatment: Date: Improvements Noticed:

_____
_____
_____
_____
_____
_____

PATIENT'S RECORD OF TREATMENTS

FOOD ITEMS: **Date Treated:** **Cleared:**

Chicken, Egg _____

Milk /Cal mix _____

Vitamin C mix _____

B. Complex Mix _____

Sugar Mix _____

Iron Mix _____

Vitamin A _____

Mineral mix _____

Salt mix/Chlorides _____

Corn mix _____

Grain mix _____

Yeast Mix/yogurt/whey _____

Art. Sweeteners _____

Coffee mix _____

Chocolate _____

Caffeine _____

Nut mix 1 _____

Nut mix 2 _____

Spice mix 1 _____

Spice mix 2 _____

Animal fat _____

Vegetable mix _____

Amino acid 1 _____

Amino acid 2 _____

Shell fish mix _____

Fish mix _____

Yogurt/Whey _____

Dried Bean mix _____

Turkey _____

Whiten-all _____

Fluoride _____

Gelatin _____

Alcohol _____
Baking powder _____
Baking soda _____
Gum mix _____
Vitamin D _____
Vitamin E _____
Vitamin K _____
Vitamin F _____
Vitamin T _____
RNA _____
DNA _____
Acid _____
Base _____
P.T. _____
Serotonin _____
Food colorings _____
Food additives _____
Cobalt _____
Copper _____
Germanium _____
Iodine _____
Lead _____
Magnesium _____
Phosphorus _____
Potassium _____
Selenium _____
Silver _____
Sulfur _____
Vanadium _____
Zinc _____
Lecithin _____
Modified Starch _____
Melon mix _____
Wheat mix _____
Potato mix _____

- Onion mix _____
- Cucumber mix _____
- Pepper mix _____
- Cheese mix _____
- Milk mix _____
- Tomato mix _____
- Vinegar mix _____
- Parasite mix _____
- Malathion _____
- Plastics _____
- Formaldehyde _____
- Crude oil _____
- Animal danders _____
- Animal epithelial _____
- Cotton mix _____
- Fabric mix _____
- Insect mix _____
- Grass mix _____
- Pollen mix _____
- Wood mix _____
- Weed mix _____
- Mold mix _____
- Dust mix _____
- Newspaper _____
- Newspaper ink _____
- Mercury _____
- Wool _____
- Tree mix _____
- Meat mix _____
- Flower mix _____
- Freon _____
- Radiation _____
- Chemicals _____
- Virus mix _____
- Bacteria mix _____

I.D. _____

Hormone _____

Smoking / cigarette _____

Perfume mix _____

Pesticides _____

Tetracycline _____

ITEMS TO TREAT TOGETHER

Certain items can be treated together if the patient is not very allergic to individual items. These items are:

1. Salt mix and chloride

2. Coffee mix, caffeine and chocolate mix

3. Nut mix 1 and nut mix 2

4. Spices 1 and spices 2

5. Yeast mix, yogurt, and whey

6. Fish mix and shell fish mix and vitamin A

7. Baking powder and baking soda

8. Newspaper and Newspaper ink

9. Animal epithelial/ Animal dander

10. Fabrics

11. Chemicals

DETAILED TREATMENT GUIDE

1. **EGG MIX.** (EGG YOLK, EGG WHITE, CHICKEN, TETRACYCLINE).

YOU MAY NOT EAT OR TOUCH: egg white, egg yolk, chicken, tetracycline and all foods containing egg or chicken including crackers, cookies, soups, breads, mayonnaise, salad dressings, cakes, pastries, pies, pancakes, foods baked or fried in egg batter and thick sauces. Also avoid birds, feather pillows, comforters, vitamins and protein drinks made with egg, shampoos, conditioners and skin lotions with egg products.

YOU MAY EAT: brown or white rice, pasta without eggs, vegetables, fruits, milk products, oils, beef, pork, fish, coffee, juice, soft drinks, water and tea.

Date treated: _____   Cleared: _____

Combinations needed: Acid/.....Base/.....DNA/.....RNA/..... Heat/......Cold/...... (RNA+DNA)=N/ .....N+Acid/......N+Base/.....N+Heat/.... N+Cold/ .. N+Acid+Heat/ N+Base+Heat/... N+Acid+Cold/ ...N+Base+Cold/..... Organs(like Lung, heart, stomach, spleen, liver, gall bladder, pancreas, kidney, small intestines, urinary bladder, colon, uterus, prostate, brain, ovary, etc.)/.....Pituitrophin/..... Serotonin/.....Hormones/.....Emotional Blockage/...Emotional Blockage +Acid/... Emotional blockage + Base / ... Emotional blockage +RNA + DNA/Emotional blockage+HEAT/ ... Emotional Blockage +COLD/ ..... Emotional Blockage + RNA+DNA/ ... Emotional Blockage +RNA+DNA+ Acid/......Emotional Blockage + RNA + DNA +BASE /.... Emotional blockage + RNA + DNA + HEAT/.... Emotional blockage + RNA + DNA + cold/... Emotional blockage + Hormone/..... Emotional blockage + Serotonin/.....Eggs + Calcium/ Eggs + Vitamin C/ Eggs + B.Complex/ Eggs + Sugar/ ... Eggs + Calcium(Milk) + B. Complex(Flour) + Sugar+Spices (Cinnamon Cookies for example.)

One may find various reactive combinations like milk & cereal, breads, cookies, ice creams, various foods and drinks. After one completes the basic ingredients, one should combine everyday foods together like breakfast, lunch & dinner of Monday, or Tuesday etc. and treat them for reaction to the food combining. In following pages, followed by each allergen, the abbreviations of the combinations are given to save space in the book.

Symptoms Noted: _____

Notes: _____
_____
_____

2. CALCIUM MIX (Cal-Carbonate, Cal- Gluconate, Cal-ascorbate, Cow's milk, goat's milk, milk-casein, milk-albumin).

YOU MAY NOT EAT OR TOUCH: milk or milk products, uncooked vegetables, dark leafy vegetables like lettuce, cabbage, dandelion greens, Brussels sprout, broccoli, sesame seeds, oats, navy beans, milk products, cheese, soybeans, almonds, dried beans, walnuts, sardines, salmon, peanuts, and sunflower seeds, calcium supplements.

YOU MAY EAT: cooked rice, cooked vegetables like potato, corn, yams, cauliflower, sweet potato, red meats, and coffee and/or tea without milk. Drink calcium- free water.

Date treated: _____   Cleared: _____

Combinations needed:..................... A/.....B/.....D/.....R/.....H/......C/.....N/..... N+A/...... N+B/.....N+H/.....N+C/.....N+A+H/.....N+B+H/.....N+A+C/.....N+B+C/.....

EB/.....EB+A/.....EB+B/.....EB+N/.....EB+H/ ...EB+C/ ..... EB+N+A/....EB+N+B/.... EB+N+A+H/....EB+N+B+H/....EB+N+A+C/...EB+N+B+C/.....

Symptoms Noted:_____

Notes:_____

3. VITAMIN C MIX (Ascorbic acid, Oxalic acid, citrus mix, berry mix, fruit mix, vegetable mix, vinegar mix, chlorophyll, hesparin, rutin, bioflavanoids).

YOU MAY NOT EAT OR TOUCH: fresh fruits, vegetables, leafy vegetables, citrus fruits, dry fruits, juices, sauces, soft drinks, milk, artificial sweeteners, and Vitamin C supplements.

YOU MAY EAT: cooked white or brown rice, pasta without sauce, boiled or poached eggs, baked or broiled chicken, fish, red meat, brown toast, deep fried food, french fries, salt, oils, and drink coffee and water.

Date treated: _____   Cleared: _____

Combinations needed:.. A/.....B/.....D/.....R/.....H/......C/.....N/..... A/......N+B/...N+H/.....N+C/.....N+A+H/...N+B+H/....N+A+C/...N+B+C/....EB/...EB+A/...EB+B/...EB+N/...EB+H/ ...EB+C/ ...EB+N+A/...EB+N+B/... +N+A+H/....EB+N+B+H/.EB+N+A+C/...EB+N+B+C/.....

Symptoms Noted:_____
Notes:_____

4. B-COMPLEX. (B1, 2, 3, 4, 5, 6, 12, 13, 15, 17, paba, inositol, choline, biotin, folic acid).

YOU MAY NOT EAT OR TOUCH: whole grain products, fruits, vegetables, meats, dairy products, anything with B vitamins.

YOU MAY EAT: cooked white rice, cauliflower raw or cooked, well cooked or deep fried fish, salt, white sugar, black coffee, french fries, and purified, non allergic water while treating for any of the B Vitamins. Rice should be washed well before cooking. Then, cook with lots of water and drain the water after cooking the rice to remove the fortified vitamins. Fish should be deep fried or well cooked.

You may refer to the following individual B-Vitamins for more information.

VITAMIN B1: (thiamine, thiamine mononitrate, thiamine chloride, thiamine HCL)

AVOID: dried yeast, rice husks, whole wheat, oatmeal, peanuts, pork, most vegetables, bran, milk, brewer's yeast, wheat germ, wheat bran, rice polishings, most whole grain cereals, milk products, leafy green vegetables, meat, liver, nuts, legumes, and potatoes.

YOU MAY EAT: white rice, white flour pasta, raw or cooked cauliflower, cooked or deep fried fish, french fries, white sugar, purified water, and black coffee.

VITAMIN B2: (riboflavin, Vitamin G)

AVOID: milk, cheese, whole grains, brewer's yeast, wheat germ, almonds, sunflower seeds, liver, cooked leafy vegetables, kidney, raw or broiled fish and eggs.

YOU MAY EAT: white rice, white flour pasta, raw or cooked cauliflower, cooked or deep fried fish, french fries, white sugar, purified water, and black coffee.

VITAMIN B3: (niacin, nicotinic acid, niacinamide)

AVOID : lean meat, raw or broiled fish, eggs, roasted peanuts, brewer's yeast, wheat germ, rice bran, rice polishings, nuts, sunflower seeds, whole wheat products, brown rice, green vegetables, liver, white meat of poultry, avocado, dates, figs, and prunes.
YOU MAY EAT: white rice, white flour pasta, raw or cooked cauliflower, cooked or deep fried fish, French fries, white sugar, purified water, and black coffee.

Vitamin B4 : (Adenine)

AVOID: whole grains, leafy vegetables, and nuts.

YOU MAY EAT: white rice, white flour pasta, raw or cooked cauliflower, cooked or deep fried fish, French fries, white sugar, purified water, and black coffee.

Vitamin B5: (pantothenic acid, calcium pantothenate)

AVOID: Brewers yeast, wheat germ, wheat bran, royal jelly, whole grain breads and cereals, green vegetables, peas, dried beans, nuts, crude molasses, raisins, cantaloupe, red meat, liver, kidney, heart, egg yolk, and chicken.

YOU MAY EAT: white rice, white flour pasta, raw or cooked cauliflower, cooked or deep fried fish, French fries, white sugar, purified water, and black coffee.

Vitamin B6: (pyridoxine, pyridoxine HCL)

AVOID: brewer's yeast, bananas, avocado, wheat germ, wheat bran, soybeans, milk, green leafy vegetables, cabbage, molasses, green peppers, legumes, cantaloupe, egg yolk, organ meats, kidney, heart, liver, and beef.

YOU MAY EAT: white rice, white flour pasta, raw or cooked cauliflower, cooked or deep fried fish, French fries, white sugar, purified water, and black coffee.

Vitamin B12: (cobalamin, cyanocobalamin)

AVOID: milk, eggs, aged cheese, yogurt, bee pollen, flower pollen, meat, liver, pork and kidney.

YOU MAY EAT: white rice, white flour pasta, raw or cooked cauliflower, cooked or deep fried fish, French fries, white sugar, purified water, and black coffee.

Vitamin B13: (orotic acid)

AVOID: milk-whey (the liquid portion of soured or curdled milk) and root vegetables.

YOU MAY EAT: white rice, white flour pasta, raw or cooked cauliflower, cooked or deep fried fish, French fries, white sugar, purified water, and black coffee.

Vitamin B15: (pangamic acid, calcium pangamate)

AVOID: whole grains, seeds, nuts, whole brown rice, brewer's yeast, pumpkin seeds and sesame seeds.

YOU MAY EAT: white rice, white flour pasta, raw or cooked cauliflower, cooked or deep fried fish, French fries, white sugar, purified water, and black coffee.

Vitamin B17: (nitrilosides, amygdalin, laetrile)

AVOID: Most whole seeds of fruits and many grains and vegetables, raspberries, cranberries, blackberries, blueberries, mung beans, lima beans, flaxseeds, whole kernels of apricots, apples, cherries, peaches, plums and nectarines.

YOU MAY EAT: white rice, white flour pasta, raw or cooked cauliflower, cooked or deep fried fish, French fries, white sugar, purified water, and black coffee.

BIOTIN: (Vitamin H, coenzyme R)

AVOID: brewer's yeast, unpolished rice, soybeans, liver, kidney, milk, molasses, nuts, fruit, beef and egg yolk.

YOU MAY EAT: white rice, white flour pasta, raw or cooked cauliflower, cooked or deep fried fish, French fries, white sugar, purified water, and black coffee.

CHOLINE:

AVOID: brewer's yeast, wheat germ, egg yolk, liver, green leafy vegetables, legumes, peas, beans, brain, heart and lecithin.

YOU MAY EAT: white rice, white flour pasta, raw or cooked cauliflower, cooked or deep fried fish, French fries, white sugar, purified water, and black coffee.

INOSITOL:

AVOID: brewer's yeast, wheat germ, lecithin, unprocessed whole grains, nuts, milk, citrus fruits, liver, dried lima beans, beef, brains, heart, raisins, cantaloupe, unrefined molasses, peanuts and cabbage.

YOU MAY EAT: white rice, white flour pasta, raw or cooked cauliflower, cooked or deep fried fish, French fries, white sugar, purified water, and black coffee.

FOLIC ACID: (Vitamin B 9, Pteroylglutamic Acid, Folate Folacin).

AVOID: dark green leafy vegetables, broccoli, asparagus, lima beans, Irish potatoes, brewer's yeast, wheat germ, mushrooms, nuts, liver, carrots, tortilla, yeast, egg yolk, cantaloupe, apricots, pumpkins, avocados, beans, whole wheat and dark rye flour.

YOU MAY EAT: white rice, white flour pasta, raw or cooked cauliflower, cooked or deep fried fish, French fries, white sugar, purified water, and black coffee.

PABA: (Para Amino Benzoic Acid, Vitamin BX)

AVOID: brewer's yeast, whole grain products, milk, eggs, yogurt, wheat germ, molasses, liver, kidney, whole grains, rice and bran.

YOU MAY EAT: white rice, white flour pasta, raw or cooked cauliflower, cooked or deep fried fish, French fries, white sugar, purified water, and black coffee.

Date treated: _____   Cleared: _____

Combinations needed:.............................. A/.....B/.....D/.....R/.....H/.......C/.....N/..... N+A/......N+B/N+H/.....N+C/.....N+A+H/.....N+B+H/.....N+A+C/.....N+B+C/.....EB/.....EB+A/.....EB+B/.....EB+N/.....EB+H/...EB+C/ ..... EB+N+A/....EB+N+B/.... B+N+A+H/EB+N+B+H/....EB+N+A+C/...EB+N+B+C/...

Symptoms Noted:_____
Notes:_____
_____

5. SUGAR MIX: (cane sugar, beet sugar, brown sugar, corn sugar, rice sugar, maple sugar, molasses, honey, fruit sugar, sucrose, glucose, dextrose, maltose, lactose, date sugar, grape sugar).

YOU MAY NOT EAT: anything with any of the above sugars, sauces, drinks with sugar. Do not use powdered spices in pre-packed containers, tooth paste and mouth washing liquids.

YOU MAY EAT: white rice, pasta, vegetables, vegetable oils, meats, eggs, chicken, water, coffee, tea without milk.

Date treated: _____   Cleared: _____

Combinations needed:.............................. A/.....B/.....D/.....R/.....H/.......C/.....N/.....
N+A/......N+B/.....N+H/.....N+C/.....N+A+H/.....N+B+H/.....N+A+C/.....N+B+C/.....
EB/.....EB+A/.....EB+B/.....EB+N/.....EB+H/ ...EB+C/ ..... EB+N+A/....EB+N+B/....
EB+N+A+H/....EB+N+B+H/....EB+N+A+C/...EB+N+B+C/.....
Symptoms Noted:_____
Notes:_____
_____

6. IRON MIX (ferrous sulfate, ferrous gluconate, beef, pork, lamb, gelatin).

YOU MAY NOT EAT OR TOUCH: apricots, peaches, banana, black molasses, dates, prunes, raisins, brewer's yeast, whole grain cereals, turnip greens, broccoli, Brussels sprout, spinach, beet tops, alfalfa, beets, sunflower seeds, walnuts, sesame seeds, whole rye, dry beans, lentils, kelp, egg yolk, red meat, pork-liver, beef, organ meats like kidney, heart and liver, farina, raw clams, oysters, nuts, asparagus, coffee, chocolate and iron supplements.

YOU MAY EAT: white rice without iron fortification, sour dough bread without iron, cauliflower, potato, chicken, light green vegetables, water and orange juice.

Date treated: _____ Cleared: _____

Combinations needed:........................... A/.....B/.....D/.....R/.....H/......C/.....N/..... N+A/......N+B/
.....N+H/.....N+C/.....N+A+H/.....N+B+H/.....N+A+C/.....N+B+C/.....

EB/.....EB+A/.....EB+B/.....EB+N/.....EB+H/ ...EB+C/ ..... EB+N+A/.....EB+N+B/.... EB+N+A+H/
....EB+N+B+H/....EB+N+A+C/...EB+N+B+C/.....

Symptoms Noted:_____

Notes:_____
_____

7. <u>VITAMIN A MIX:</u> FISH, SHELL FISH MIX

(beta carotene, vitamin A, fish, shell fish sources).

YOU MAY NOT USE OR TOUCH: yellow fruits, yellow vegetables, green fruits, green vegetables, green peppers, fish or fish products, milk products and corn products.

YOU MAY USE: steamed rice, pasta, potato, cauliflower, red apples, chicken, water and coffee.

Date treated: _____ Cleared: _____

Combinations needed:........................... A/.....B/.....D/.....R/.....H/......C/.....N/..... N+A/......N+B/
.....N+H/.....N+C/.....N+A+H/.....N+B+H/.....N+A+C/.....N+B+C/.....

EB/.....EB+A/.....EB+B/.....EB+N/.....EB+H/ ...EB+C/ ..... EB+N+A/.....EB+N+B/.... EB+N+A+H/
....EB+N+B+H/....EB+N+A+C/...EB+N+B+C/.....

Symptoms Noted:_____

Notes:_____
_____

8. MINERAL MIX (trace minerals like antimony, barium, boron, beryllium, bromide, caesium, chlorine, chromium, cobalt, copper, europium, fluorine, gallium, germanium, gold, iodine, lithium, manganese, molybdenum, nickel, palladium, rubidium, samarium, scandium, silver, strontium, thallium, thorium, tin, titanium, tungsten, uranium, zinc, zirconium, chromium, lead, magnesium, manganese, phosphorus, potassium, selenium, sulfur, vanadium, mercury).

YOU MAY NOT USE OR TOUCH: metals, tap water, mineral water, root vegetables like onion, potato, carrots and turnips. Wear gloves while touching metal surfaces. Metal buttons on clothes, shoes, hand bags, wedding rings or religious rings, etc. can be covered with masking tape. Use plastic and glass utensils to cook and eat. Use a pair of gloves during 25 hour period to avoid touching metals.

YOU MAY USE: distilled water for washing and showering, steamed rice, vegetables, fruits, meats, eggs, milk, coffee and tea.

Date treated:_____ Cleared: _____

Combinations needed:............................. A/.....B/.....D/.....R/.....H/.......C/.....N/..... N+A/.......N+B/
.....N+H/.....N+C/.....N+A+H/.....N+B+H/.....N+A+C/.....N+B+C/.....

EB/.....EB+A/.....EB+B/.....EB+N/.....EB+H/ ...EB+C/ ..... EB+N+A/....EB+N+B/... EB+N+A+H/
....EB+N+B+H/....EB+N+A+C/...EB+N+B+C/.....

Symptoms Noted:_____
Notes: _____
_____

9. SALT MIX, CHLORIDES: (sea salt, table salt, rock salt, sodium and chloride).

YOU MAY NOT USE OR TOUCH: kelp, celery, romaine lettuce, watermelon, sea food, processed foods with salt, fast foods, table salt, fish, shell fish, carrots, beets, artichoke, dried beef, brain, kidney, cured meats, bacon, ham, coffee, watercress, sea weed, oats, avocado, Swiss chard, tomatoes, cabbage, cucumber, asparagus, pineapple, tap water, and prepared , canned or frozen foods.

YOU MAY USE: distilled water to drink and bathe, steamed rice, fresh vegetables and fruits not listed above, chicken, meats and sugars.

Date treated: _____ Cleared: _____

The NAET Guide Book

Combinations needed:............................. A/.....B/.....D/.....R/.....H/......C/..... N/..... N+A/.....
N+B/.....N+H/.....N+C/.....N+A+H/.....N+B+H/.....N+A+C/.....N+B+C/.....EB/.....EB+A/.....
EB+B/.....EB+N/.....EB+H/ ...EB+C/ ..... EB+N+A/....EB+N+B/ .... B+N+A+H/....
EB+N+B+H/....EB+N+A+C/...EB+N+B+C/.....

Symptoms Noted: _____
Notes:_____

10. CORN MIX: (blue corn, yellow corn, white corn, cornstarch, cornsilk, corn syrup).

AVOID: corn starch and any food prepared with corn starch and oil such as sauces, syrups, corn syrups, soft drinks, carbonated drinks, breads, creams. Also avoid shampoos, tooth paste, baking soda, baking powder, and deodorants.

YOU MAY USE: steamed vegetables, steamed rice, broccoli, baked chicken, and meats. You may drink water, tea and/or coffee without cream or sugar.

Date treated: _____ Cleared: _____

Combinations needed:............................. A/.....B/.....D/.....R/.....H/......C/.....N/....
N+A/......N+B/.....N+H/.....N+C/.....N+A+H/.....N+B+H/.....N+A+C/.....N+B+C/....
EB/.....EB+A/.....EB+B/.....EB+N/.....EB+H/ ...EB+C/ ..... EB+N+A/....EB+N+B/EB+N+A+H/....EB+N+B+H/....EB+N+A+C/...EB+N+B+C/.....

Symptoms Noted:_____
Notes:_____
_____

11. GRAIN MIX: (wheat, corn, rice, oats, rye, millet, barley).

YOU MAY NOT USE: grains and items made from above grains.

YOU MAY EAT: vegetables, fruits, meats, milk and drink water.

Date treated: _____ Cleared: _____

Combinations needed:... A/.....B/.....D/.....R/.....H/......C/
EB/.....EB+A/.....EB+B/.....EB+N/.....EB+H/ ...EB+C/ ..... EB+N+A/....EB+N+B/.... EB+N+A+H/
....EB+N+B+H/....EB+N+A+C/...EB+N+B+C/.....

Symptoms Noted:_____
Notes:_____
_____

12. ARTIFICIAL SWEETENERS: (Equal, Nutrasweet, Aspartame, Sorbitol, Sweet And Low, Twin and Saccharine).

AVOID: items with the above artificial sugars, like soft drinks, sweet relish, pickles, sauces, cookies, tooth paste, mouthwash, etc.

YOU MAY EAT: anything without artificial sweeteners. Use freshly prepared items only.

Date treated: _____ Cleared: _____

Combinations needed:............................... A/.....B/.....D/.....R/.....H/......C/.....
N/.....N+A/......N+B/.....N+H/.....N+C/.....N+A+H/.....N+B+H/.....N+A+C/.....
N+B+C/..... EB/.....EB+A/.....EB+B/.....EB+N/.....EB+H/ ...EB+C/ .....
EB+N+A/....EB+N+B/....EB+N+A+H/....EB+N+B+H/....EB+N+A+C/...
EB+N+B+C/.....

Symptoms Noted:_____
Notes:_____
_____

13. COFFEE MIX: Coffee, Chocolate mix, caffeine, tea, tannic acid, cocoa, cocoa butter, carob.

YOU MAY NOT USE OR SMELL: Coffee, tea, caffeinated drinks, leather goods, tannic acids, chocolate and all foods containing chocolate, like ice cream, coffee and tea.

YOU MAY EAT: anything that has no coffee, caffeine or chocolate.

Date treated: _____ Cleared: _____

Combinations needed:.. A/...B/...D/...R/...H/...C/...N/...N+A/...N+B/... N+H/...N+C/... N+A+H/...N+B+H/...N+A+C/... N+B+C/... EB/...EB+A/...EB+B/... EB+N/...EB+H/... EB+C/ ... EB+N+A/...EB+N+B/...EB+N+A+H/...EB+N+B+H/... EB+N+A+C/... EB+N+B+C/...

Symptoms Noted:_____

Notes:_____

_____

14. NUT MIX 1 (peanuts, black walnut, English walnut).

YOU MAY NOT EAT OR TOUCH: peanuts, walnuts, black walnuts, and English walnuts or anything made from these nuts or their oils.

YOU MAY EAT: any foods that do not contain the nuts listed above including their oils and butters.

Date treated: _____ Cleared: _____

Combinations needed:.. A/...B/...D/...R/...H/...C/...N/...N+A/...N+B/...N+H/...N+C/.....N+A+H/.....N+B+H/.....N+A+C/...N+B+C/...EB/...EB+A/...EB+B/...EB+N/... EB+H/ ...EB+C/ ... EB+N+A/...EB+N+B/...EB+N+A+H/... EB+N+B+H/....EB+N+A+C/...EB+N+B+C/.....

Symptoms Noted:_____
Notes:_____

_____

15. NUT MIX 2 (cashew, almonds, pecan, Brazil nut, hazelnut, macadamia, sunflower seeds).

YOU MAY NOT EAT OR TOUCH: any of the above mentioned nuts or oils.

YOU MAY EAT: any foods that do not contain the nuts listed above including their oils and butters.

Date treated:_____ Cleared: _____

Combinations needed:.. A/...B/...D/...R/...H/...C/...N/...N+A/....N+B/...
N+H/.....N+C/.....N+A+H/.....N+B+H/.....N+A+C/.....N+B+C/.....
EB/.....EB+A/.....EB+B/.....EB+N/.....EB+H/ ...EB+C/ ..... EB+N+A/....EB+N+B/....
EB+N+A+H/....EB+N+B+H/....EB+N+A+C/...EB+N+B+C/.....

Symptoms Noted:_____

Notes:_____

_____

16. SPICE MIX 1 (ginger, cardamom, cinnamon, cloves, nutmeg, garlic, cumin, fennel, coriander, turmeric, saffron, mint).

AVOID: above listed spices in any form. These spices and their oils are encountered in candies, chewing gums, tooth paste, massage oils, aroma therapy ingredients and toiletries.

YOU MAY USE: all foods, and products without these items.

Date treated: _____ Cleared: _____

combinations needed:.. A/...B/...D/...R/...H/....C/...N/...N+A/...N+B/...N+H/...
N+C/...N+A+H/...N+B+H/...N+A+C/...N+B+C/...EB/...EB+A/...EB+B/...
EB+N/...EB+H/ ...EB+C/... EB+N+A/...EB+N+B/...EB+N+A+H/...
EB+N+B+H/...EB+N+A+C/...EB+N+B+C/...

Symptoms Noted: _____

Notes:_____

_____

17. SPICE MIX 2 (peppers, red pepper, black pepper, green pepper, jalapino, banana peppers, anise seed, basil, bay leaf, caraway seed, chervil, cream of tartar, dill, fenugreek, horseradish, mace, MSG, mustard, onion, oregano, paprika, poppy seed, parsley, rosemary, sage, sumac, and vinegar).

AVOID: any of the above spices.

YOU MAY USE: all foods and food products without the above listed spices.

Date treated: _____Cleared: _____

Combinations needed:... A/...B/...D/...R/...H/...C/...N/...N+A/....N+B/...N+H/...
N+C/...N+A+H/...N+B+H/...N+A+C/...N+B+C/...EB/...EB+A/...EB+B/...
EB+N/.....EB+H/ ...EB+C/ ..... EB+N+A/....EB+N+B/...EB+N+A+H/...
EB+N+B+H/...EB+N+A+C/...EB+N+B+C/....

Symptoms Noted:_____
Notes:_____
_____

18. ANIMAL FAT: (butter, lard, chicken fat, beef fat, lamb fat, fish oil).

YOU MAY NOT USE OR TOUCH: butter, lard, meats, fish and fish oils, skin lotions with lanolin or animal fat, food fried in animal fat, refried beans, chili beans, corn chips fried in lard etc.

YOU MAY USE: anything other than the above including vegetable oils.

Date treated: _____ Cleared: _____

Combinations needed:... A/...B/...D/...R/...H/....C/...N/...N+A/...N+B/...N+H/...
N+C/...N+A+H/...N+B+H/...N+A+C/...N+B+C/...EB/...EB+A/...EB+B/...
EB+N/...EB+H/ ...EB+C/ ... EB+N+A/...EB+N+B/...EB+N+A+H/...
EB+N+B+H/...EB+N+A+C/...EB+N+B+C/...

Symptoms Noted:_____
Notes:_____
_____

19. **VEGETABLE FATS:** (Corn oil, canola oil, peanut oil, linseed oil, sun flower oil, palm oil, flax seed oil, coconut oil).

YOU MAY NOT USE: vegetable oils, foods containing vegetable oils like breads, crackers, cookies, sauces, drinks, and skin lotions, makeup items, shampoo, conditioner, etc.

YOU MAY USE: steamed vegetables, steamed rice, meats, eggs, chicken, butter and animal fats.

Date treated: _____ Cleared: _____

Combinations needed:.... A/...B/...D/...R/...H/....C/...N/...N+A/....N+B/...
N+H/...N+C/...N+A+H/...N+B+H/...N+A+C/...N+B+C/...EB/...EB+A/...
EB+B/...EB+N/...EB+H/ ...EB+C/ .... EB+N+A/...EB+N+B/...
EB+N+A+H/...EB+N+B+H/...EB+N+A+C/... EB+N+B+C/...

Symptoms Noted:_____
Notes:_____
_____

20. **AMINO ACIDS 1 & 11:** (essential amino acids: Lysine, methionine, leucine, threonine, Valine, thryptophane, isoleucine, and phenylalanine, non essential amino acids: alanine, arginine, aspartic acid, carnitine, citrulline, cysteine, glutathione, glutamic acid, glycine, histidine, ornithine, proline, serine, taurine, tyrosine).

YOU MAY NOT EAT OR TOUCH: any type of food that contains proteins, and protein products that are used for external application.

YOU MAY EAT: steamed white rice, lettuce and drink water.

Date treated:_____ Cleared: _____

Combinations needed:.. A/...B/...D/...R/...H/...C/...N/...N+A/...N+B/...N+H/...N+C/... N+A+H/...N+B+H/ ...N+A+C/...N+B+C/...EB/...EB+A/...EB+B/...EB+N/...
EB+H/...EB+C/...EB+N+A/...EB+N+B/...EB+N+A+H/...EB+N+B+H/.... EB+N+A+C/... EB+N+B+C/.....

Symptoms Noted:_____
Notes:_____
_____

21. FISH MIX: (Cod, Halibut, Salmon, Tuna, Shark).

YOU MAY NOT EAT OR SMELL tuna, salmon, halibut, cod, their oils, and glues on the stamps, envelopes, and anything else made from fish source.

YOU MAY EAT any food that does not contain the fish or fish oils listed above.

Date treated: _____ Cleared: _____

Combinations needed:.. A/...B/...D/...R/...H/...C/...N/...N+A/...N+B/...N+H/...
N+C/...N+A+H/...N+B+H/...N+A+C/...N+B+C/...EB/...EB+A/...EB+B/...
EB+N/...EB+H/ ...EB+C/ ... EB+N+A/...EB+N+B/...EB+N+A+H/...
EB+N+B+H/...EB+N+A+C/...EB+N+B+C/...

Symptoms Noted:_____
Notes:_____
_____

22. SHELLFISH MIX: (Shrimp, lobster, abalone, cray, crab, clams).

YOU MAY NOT EAT OR SMELL any fish or fish products.

YOU MAY EAT any food that does not contain fish products.

Date treated: _____ Cleared: _____

Combinations needed:.. A/...B/...D/...R/...H/...C/...N/...N+A/...N+B/...N+H/...
N+C/...N+A+H/...N+B+H/...N+A+C/...N+B+C/...EB/...EB+A/...EB+B/...
EB+N/...EB+H/ ...EB+C/ ... EB+N+A/...EB+N+B/...EB+N+A+H/...
EB+N+B+H/...EB+N+A+C/...EB+N+B+C/...

Symptoms Noted:_____
Notes:_____

23. YEAST MIX: (Baker's Yeast, Brewer's Yeast, Tortula Yeast).

AVOID: Brewer's yeast, bakers yeast, and any foods containing these items including baked goods, sugars, fruits, soy sauce, and alcoholic beverages.

YOU MAY EAT vegetables, meat, chicken and fish.

Date treated: _____ Cleared: _____

Combinations needed:.. A/...B/...D/...R/...H/...C/...N/...N+A/...N+B/...N+H/...N+C/... N+A+H/...N+B+H/...N+A+C/...N+B+C/...EB/...EB+A/...EB+B/...EB+N/...
EB+H/...EB+C/...EB+N+A/...EB+N+B/...EB+N+A+H/...EB+N+B+H/.... EB+N+A+C/... EB+N+B+C/.....

Symptoms Noted:_____
Notes:_____
_____

24. WHEY:

AVOID: Cottage cheese, all yogurts and items made with whey like crackers, french breads, yogurt or cheese.

YOU MAY EAT rice, vegetables, fruits, chicken, egg, turkey, beef, pork, beans, and lamb.

Treated: _____ Cleared: _____

Combinations needed:.. A/...B/...D/...R/...H/...C/...N/...N+A/...N+B/...N+H/...N+C/... N+A+H/...N+B+H/...N+A+C/...N+B+C/...EB/...EB+A/...EB+B/...EB+N/...
EB+H/...EB+C/...EB+N+A/...EB+N+B/...EB+N+A+H/...EB+N+B+H/.... EB+N+A+C/... EB+N+B+C/.....

Symptoms Noted:_____
Notes:_____
_____

25. YOGURT

AVOID: cottage cheese, all yogurts, and items made with whey, yogurt or cheese.

YOU MAY EAT rice, vegetables, fruits, poultry, and meat.

Date treated: _____ Cleared: _____

Combinations needed:.. A/...B/...D/...R/...H/...C/...N/...N+A/...N+B/...N+H/...N+C/... N+A+H/...N+B+H/...N+A+C/...N+B+C/...EB/...EB+A/...EB+B/...EB+N/...

EB+H/...EB+C/...EB+N+A/...EB+N+B/...EB+N+A+H/...EB+N+B+H/.... EB+N+A+C/... EB+N+B+C/.....

Symptoms Noted:_____

Notes:_____

_____

26. DRIED BEANS MIX : (Pinto beans, lima beans, lentils, peas, garbanzo beans, black beans, red beans, black eye peas, navy beans).

AVOID: above listed beans, their oils or products.

YOU MAY EAT anything other than beans or bean products (rice, pasta, vegetables, meats, eggs, etc.).

Date treated: _____ Cleared: _____

Combinations needed:.. A/...B/...D/...R/...H/...C/...N/...N+A/...N+B/...N+H/...N+C/... N+A+H/...N+B+H/...N+A+C/...N+B+C/...EB/...EB+A/...EB+B/...EB+N/...

EB+H/...EB+C/...EB+N+A/...EB+N+B/...EB+N+A+H/...EB+N+B+H/.... EB+N+A+C/... EB+N+B+C/...

Symptoms Noted:_____

Notes:_____

_____

27. TURKEY: (turkey, serotonin).

AVOID: Turkey in any form, milk products, tryptophane, vitamin B1, B3 and B6 and all the products with these vitamins (vitamin B1, B3, B6, tryptophane are the precursors of serotonin).

YOU MAY EAT any food that does not contain the above listed items.

Date treated: _____   Cleared: _____

Combinations needed:.. A/...B/...D/...R/...H/...C/...N/...N+A/...N+B/...N+H/...N+C/... N+A+H/...N+B+H/...N+A+C/...N+B+C/...EB/...EB+A/...EB+B/...EB+N/...

EB+H/...EB+C/...EB+N+A/...EB+N+B/...EB+N+A+H/...EB+N+B+H/.... EB+N+A+C/... EB+N+B+C/.....

Symptoms Noted:_____

Notes:_____

_____

_____

28. WHITEN-ALL

AVOID: Uncooked vegetables, fresh fruits, frozen vegetables, canned foods, potato salads, fruit salads made at the restaurant, or pre packed by catering companies, French fries, baked potato, any other potato prepared by caterers, sauces, dips, etc.

YOU MAY EAT Cooked vegetables, pasta, rice, meats, chicken and eggs.

Date treated: _____   Cleared: _____

Combinations needed:.. A/...B/...D/...R/...H/...C/...N/...N+A/...N+B/...N+H/...N+C/... N+A+H/...N+B+H/...N+A+C/...N+B+C/...EB/...EB+A/...EB+B/...EB+N/...

EB+H/...EB+C/...EB+N+A/...EB+N+B/...EB+N+A+H/...EB+N+B+H/.... EB+N+A+C/... EB+N+B+C/.....

Symptoms Noted:_____

Notes:_____

_____

29. FLUORIDE

AVOID: Fluoridated water, gelatin, sunflower seeds, milk, cheese, carrots, garlic, almonds, green leafy vegetables and fish. Do not bathe in or drink fluoridated water. Do not eat products prepared with sunflower oil.

YOU MAY USE OR EAT fruits, poultry, meat, potato, cauliflower, white rice, and yellow vegetables. If you are also treating for water you may drink fresh fruit juices, and distilled water.

Date treated: _____ Cleared: _____

Combinations needed:.. A/...B/...D/...R/...H/...C/...N/...N+A/...N+B/...N+H/...N+C/...
N+A+H/...N+B+H/...N+A+C/...N+B+C/...EB/...EB+A/...EB+B/...EB+N/...EB+H/...
EB+C/...EB+N+A/...EB+N+B/...EB+N+A+H/...EB+N+B+H/.... EB+N+A+C/... EB+N+B+C/.....
Symptoms Noted:_____
Notes:_____
_____

30. GELATIN

AVOID: Apple skin, pectin, hard skin of other fruits, okra, gelatin from chicken, meat, gelatin capsules, Jell-O, gelatin- added puddings, sticky candy, cosmetics, facial masks, and other makeup products.

YOU MAY USE the things that do not contain gelatin.

Date treated: _____ Cleared: _____

Combinations needed:.. A/...B/...D/...R/...H/...C/...N/...N+A/...N+B/...N+H/...N+C/...
N+A+H/...N+B+H/...N+A+C/...N+B+C/...EB/...EB+A/...EB+B/...EB+N/...EB+H/...
EB+C/...EB+N+A/...EB+N+B/...EB+N+A+H/...EB+N+B+H/.... EB+N+A+C/... EB+N+B+C/.....
Symptoms Noted:_____
Notes:_____
_____

31. ALCOHOL: (beer, red wine, white wine, rubbing alcohol, cooking wine, champagne, tequila and vodka.)

AVOID : All alcoholic beverages, vanilla ice cream, foods cooked with wine, sugar and starchy foods, fruits, hair sprays, medicine with alcohols like cough syrups, shampoos, hair products, cosmetics and makeup products and rubbing alcohols.

YOU MAY USE Things not listed above. May eat vegetables, meats, fish, eggs and chicken.

Date treated: _____ Cleared: _____

Combinations needed:.. A/...B/...D/...R/...H/...C/...N/...N+A/...N+B/...N+H/...N+C/... N+A+H/...N+B+H/...N+A+C/...N+B+C/...EB/...EB+A/...EB+B/...EB+N/...

EB+H/...EB+C/...EB+N+A/...EB+N+B/...EB+N+A+H/...EB+N+B+H/.... EB+N+A+C/... EB+N+B+C/.....

Symptoms Noted: _____
Notes: _____
_____

32. BAKING POWDER/ BAKING SODA

AVOID: Baking powder, baking soda, and foods, medications and tooth pastes, deodorants, antiperspirants, talcum powders, soaps, detergents and cotton crotches of female underpants containing baking soda.

YOU MAY EAT OR USE any foods which do not contain the items listed above including fresh fruits, vegetables, fats, meat and chicken.

Date treated: _____ Cleared: _____

33. GUM MIX: Acacia, Karaya gum, Xanthine gum, Black gum, Sweet gum and chewing gum.

AVOID : Soft drinks, glues, chewing gum, cream cheese, and carbonated drinks. Please read the labels on the food containers if you are buying from the market.

YOU MAY USE things not containing gums. You may eat rice, pasta, vegetables, fruits without skins, meats, eggs and chicken.

Date treated: _____ Cleared: _____

Combinations needed:............ A/.....B/.....D/.....R/.....H/.......C/.....N/.....N+A/......N+B/....N+H/.....N+C/.....N+A+H/.....N+B+H/.....N+A+C/.....N+B+C/.....EB/.....EB+A/.....EB+B/.....EB+N/.....EB+H/ ...EB+C/ ..... EB+N+A/....EB+N+B/.

...EB+N+A+H/....EB+N+B+H/....EB+N+A+C/...EB+N+B+C/.....

Symptoms Noted:_____

Notes:_____

_____

34. VITAMIN E

(Tocopherol, d-Alpha Tocopherol, or Tocopheryl, D1-Alpha Tocopherol, or Tocopheryl, Mixed Tocopherols).

AVOID: Wheat germ, soybeans, vegetable oils, broccoli, brussels sprout, leafy greens, spinach, enriched flour, whole wheat, whole grain cereals, eggs, unrefined cold pressed crude vegetable oils, wheat germ and soybean oils, whole, raw or sprouted seeds, nuts and grains.

YOU MAY EAT fresh fruit, carrots, potatoes, poultry and meat.

Date treated: _____ Cleared: _____

Combinations needed:.. A/...B/...D/...R/...H/...C/...N/...N+A/...N+B/...N+H/...N+C/... N+A+H/...N+B+H/...N+A+C/...N+B+C/...EB/...EB+A/...EB+B/...EB+N/...

EB+H/...EB+C/...EB+N+A/...EB+N+B/...EB+N+A+H/...EB+N+B+H/.... EB+N+A+C/... EB+N+B+C/ .....

Symptoms Noted:_____

Notes:_____

_____

35. VITAMIN D: (Ergosterol, Viosterol, Calciferol, Cholecalciferol or Cholecalciferol, Ergocalciferol, Sunshine Vitamin).

AVOID: Fish liver oil, egg yolks, milk, butter, sprouted seeds, mushrooms, sunflower seeds and sunflower oil.

YOU MAY EAT any foods not listed above including fruits, vegetables, poultry and meat.

Date treated: _____ Cleared: _____

Combinations needed:.. A/...B/...D/...R/...H/...C/...N/...N+A/...N+B/...N+H/...N+C/... N+A+H/...N+B+H/...N+A+C/...N+B+C/...EB/...EB+A/...EB+B/...EB+N/...
EB+H/...EB+C/...EB+N+A/...EB+N+B/...EB+N+A+H/...EB+N+B+H/.... EB+N+A+C/... EB+N+B+C/.....

Symptoms Noted: _____
Notes: _____
_____

36. VITAMIN K: (phytomenadione, phytonadione, phylloquinone, menadione).

AVOID : Kelp, alfalfa and other green plants, soybean oils, egg yolks, cow's milk, liver, yogurt, safflower and soybean oils, fish liver oils, cabbage, Brussels sprout and green leafy vegetable.

YOU MAY EAT : Fruit, rice, potato, poultry and meat.

Date treated: _____ Cleared : _____

Combinations needed:.. A/...B/...D/...R/...H/...C/...N/...N+A/...N+B/...N+H/...N+C/... N+A+H/...N+B+H/...N+A+C/...N+B+C/...EB/...EB+A/...EB+B/...EB+N/...
EB+H/...EB+C/...EB+N+A/...EB+N+B/...EB+N+A+H/...EB+N+B+H/.... EB+N+A+C/... EB+N+B+C/.....

Symptoms Noted: _____
Notes: _____
_____

37. **VITAMIN F:** (Unsaturated fatty acids-linoleic, gamma-linoleic and arachinoidic factors).

AVOID: Vegetable oils, wheat germ oils, linseed oils, sunflower oils, safflower oils, soybean oils, peanuts and peanut oils, flax seeds, evening primrose oils, all nuts and breast milk.

YOU MAY EAT anything that is not in the above list

Date treated:_____ Cleared:_____

Combinations needed:.. A/...B/...D/...R/...H/...C/...N/...N+A/...N+B/...N+H/...N+C/... N+A+H/...N+B+H/...N+A+C/...N+B+C/...EB/...EB+A/...EB+B/...EB+N/...
EB+H/...EB+C/...EB+N+A/...EB+N+B/...EB+N+A+H/...EB+N+B+H/.... EB+N+A+C/...EB+N+B+C/.....

Symptoms Noted:_____
Notes:_____
_____

38. **VITAMIN P:** (Bioflavanoids, citrus bioflavonoids, hesperidin, rutin). This is very essential for venous and capillary integrity.

AVOID: Rose hips, buckwheat, citrus fruit pulp, green peppers, grapes, apricot, strawberries, black currants, cherries, prunes, white skin and segment part of citrus fruit, oranges, grapefruit, lemons and black berries.

YOU MAY EAT things not in the above list.

Date treated:_____ Cleared:_____

Combinations needed:.. A/...B/...D/...R/...H/...C/...N/...N+A/...N+B/...N+H/...N+C/... N+A+H/...N+B+H/...N+A+C/...N+B+C/...EB/...EB+A/...EB+B/...EB+N/...
EB+H/...EB+C/...EB+N+A/...EB+N+B/...EB+N+A+H/...EB+N+B+H/.... EB+N+A+C/... EB+N+B+C/.....

Symptoms Noted:_____
Notes:_____
_____

39. VITAMIN T: (sesame seed factor).

AVOID: sesame seeds, egg yolks, vegetable oils.

YOU MAY EAT anything other than in the above list.

Date treated:_____ Cleared: _____

Combinations needed:.. A/...B/...D/...R/...H/...C/...N/...N+A/...N+B/...N+H/...N+C/... N+A+H/...N+B+H/...N+A+C/...N+B+C/...EB/...EB+A/...EB+B/...EB+N/...
EB+H/...EB+C/...EB+N+A/...EB+N+B/...EB+N+A+H/...EB+N+B+H/.... EB+N+A+C/... EB+N+B+C/.....

Symptoms Noted: _____

Notes:_____

_____

40. RNA/DNA

AVOID: All type of proteins.

YOU MAY EAT white rice and lettuce.

Date treated: _____ Cleared: _____

Combinations needed:.. A/...B/...D/...R/...H/...C/...N/...N+A/...N+B/...N+H/...N+C/... N+A+H/...N+B+H/...N+A+C/...N+B+C/...EB/...EB+A/...EB+B/...EB+N/...
EB+H/...EB+C/...EB+N+A/...EB+N+B/...EB+N+A+H/...EB+N+B+H/.... EB+N+A+C/... EB+N+B+C/.....

Symptoms Noted:_____

Notes:_____

_____

41. STOMACH ACIDS

AVOID : Sugar, starches, fruits, grains, meats, other acid forming foods.

YOU MAY EAT raw and steamed vegetables, cooked dried beans, eggs, oils, clarified butter, and milk.

Date treated:_____ Cleared :_____

Combinations needed:.. A/...B/...D/...R/...H/...C/...N/...N+A/...N+B/...N+H/...N+C/... N+A+H/...N+B+H/...N+A+C/...N+B+C/...EB/...EB+A/...EB+B/...EB+N/...
EB+H/...EB+C/...EB+N+A/...EB+N+B/...EB+N+A+H/...EB+N+B+H/.... EB+N+A+C/... EB+N+B+C/.....

Symptoms Noted:_____
Notes:_____
_____

42. BASE: (Digestive juices and enzymes from intestinal tracts).

AVOID : Raw and cooked vegetables, beans , eggs, and milk.

YOU MAY EAT sugars, starches, breads and meats.

Date treated:_____Cleared:_____

Combinations needed:.. A/...B/...D/...R/...H/...C/...N/...N+A/...N+B/...N+H/...N+C/... N+A+H/...N+B+H/...N+A+C/...N+B+C/...EB/...EB+A/...EB+B/...EB+N/...
EB+H/...EB+C/...EB+N+A/...EB+N+B/...EB+N+A+H/...EB+N+B+H/.... EB+N+A+C/... EB+N+B+C/.....

Symptoms Noted:_____
Notes:_____
_____

43. FOOD COLORING

AVOID colored foods, pre mixed powdered spices, frozen vegetables, sauces, candies, chewing gums, soft drinks, ice creams, lipstick, crayons, coloring books, etc.

YOU MAY EAT fresh vegetables, rice, pasta, eggs, chicken, milk and water.

Date treated:_____ Cleared:_____

Combinations needed:.. A/...B/...D/...R/...H/...C/...N/...N+A/...N+B/...N+H/...N+C/... N+A+H/...N+B+H/...N+A+C/...N+B+C/...EB/...EB+A/...EB+B/...EB+N/...
EB+H/...EB+C/...EB+N+A/...EB+N+B/...EB+N+A+H/...EB+N+B+H/.... EB+N+A+C/... EB+N+B+C/.....

Symptoms Noted:_____
Notes:_____
_____

44. FOOD ADDITIVES: (Sodium nitrates, sodium phosphates, calcium sulfates, calcium phosphates).

AVOID : Hot dogs, sausages, pre-packed meats, soups, crackers, certain cookies (read labels), salad dressings, sauces etc.

YOU MAY EAT : Fresh vegetables, freshly cooked grains, eggs, chicken and milk.

Date treated:_____ Cleared:_____

Combinations needed:.. A/...B/...D/...R/...H/...C/...N/...N+A/...N+B/...N+H/...N+C/... N+A+H/...N+B+H/...N+A+C/...N+B+C/...EB/...EB+A/...EB+B/...EB+N/...
EB+H/...EB+C/...EB+N+A/...EB+N+B/...EB+N+A+H/...EB+N+B+H/.... EB+N+A+C/... EB+N+B+C/.....

Symptoms Noted:_____
Notes:_____
_____

The following items are included in the mineral mix. After you clear the mineral mix, you must check these individually.

45. CHROMIUM

AVOID: Whole grains, wheat germ, corn oil, brewers yeast, mushrooms, meat, liver, sugar, shellfish, clams, chicken.

YOU MAY EAT: White rice and pasta, cauliflower, potato, fruits, table salt, drink water.

Date treated:_____ Cleared: _____

Combinations needed:.. A/...B/...D/...R/...H/...C/...N/...N+A/...N+B/...N+H/...N+C/... N+A+H/...N+B+H/ ...N+A+C/...N+B+C/...EB/...EB+A/...EB+B/...EB+N/...
EB+H/...EB+C/...EB+N+A/...EB+N+B/...EB+N+A+H/...EB+N+B+H/.... EB+N+A+C/... EB+N+B+C/ .....

46. COBALT

AVOID: Green leafy vegetables, meat, liver, kidney, figs, buckwheat, oyster, clams, milk.

YOU MAY EAT: white rice and pasta, cauliflower, potato, fresh fruits, non iodized salt, drink water.

Date treated:_____ Cleared: _____

Combinations needed:.. A/...B/...D/...R/...H/...C/...N/...N+A/...N+B/...N+H/...N+C/... N+A+H/...N+B+H/ ...N+A+C/...N+B+C/...EB/...EB+A/...EB+B/...EB+N/...
EB+H/...EB+C/...EB+N+A/...EB+N+B/...EB+N+A+H/...EB+N+B+H/.... EB+N+A+C/... EB+N+B+C/ .....

Symptoms Noted:_____
Notes:_____
_____

47. COPPER

AVOID almonds, green beans, peas, green leafy vegetables, whole grains, prunes, raisins, liver, dried beans, whole wheat, beef liver, calf liver, shrimp, seafood.

YOU MAY EAT white rice and pasta, cauliflower, potato, fresh fruits, non iodized salt, drink water.

Date treated:_____ Cleared: _____

Combinations needed:.. A/...B/...D/...R/...H/...C/...N/...N+A/...N+B/...N+H/...N+C/... N+A+H/...N+B+H/...N+A+C/...N+B+C/...EB/...EB+A/...EB+B/...EB+N/...
EB+H/...EB+C/...EB+N+A/...EB+N+B/...EB+N+A+H/...EB+N+B+H/.... EB+N+A+C/... EB+N+B+C/.....

Symptoms Noted:_____
Notes:_____

48. GERMANIUM

AVOID all whole grains and sprouts including breads.

YOU MAY EAT fruit, vegetables, vegetable oils, dairy, poultry and meats.

Date treated:_____ Cleared: _____

Combinations needed:.. A/...B/...D/...R/...H/...C/...N/...N+A/...N+B/...N+H/...N+C/... N+A+H/...N+B+H/...N+A+C/...N+B+C/...EB/...EB+A/...EB+B/...EB+N/...
EB+H/...EB+C/...EB+N+A/...EB+N+B/...EB+N+A+H/...EB+N+B+H/.... EB+N+A+C/... EB+N+B+C/.....

Symptoms Noted:_____
Notes:_____

49. IODINE

AVOID kelp, seafood, iodized salt, onions.

YOU MAY EAT rice and pasta, cauliflower, potato, fruits, non iodized salt, drink water.

Date treated:_____ Cleared:_____

Combinations needed:.. A/...B/...D/...R/...H/...C/...N/...N+A/...N+B/...N+H/...N+C/... N+A+H/...N+B+H/...N+A+C/...N+B+C/...EB/...EB+A/...EB+B/...EB+N/...
EB+H/...EB+C/...EB+N+A/...EB+N+B/...EB+N+A+H/...EB+N+B+H/.... EB+N+A+C/... EB+N+B+C/.....

Symptoms Noted:_____
Notes:_____

50. MAGNESIUM

AVOID nuts, soybeans, raw and cooked green leafy vegetables, almonds, whole grains, sunflower seeds, brown rice, sesame seeds.

YOU MAY EAT white rice, potato, cauliflower, eggs, chicken, meats, milk and fruits.

Date treated:_____ Cleared:_____

Combinations needed:.. A/...B/...D/...R/...H/...C/...N/...N+A/...N+B/...N+H/...N+C/... N+A+H/...N+B+H/...N+A+C/...N+B+C/...EB/...EB+A/...EB+B/...EB+N/...
EB+H/...EB+C/...EB+N+A/...EB+N+B/...EB+N+A+H/...EB+N+B+H/.... EB+N+A+C/... EB+N+B+C/.....

Symptoms Noted:_____
Notes:_____

51. MANGANESE

AVOID green leafy vegetables, beets, blueberries, oranges, grapefruit, apricot, the outer coating of nuts and grains (bran), peas, kelp, raw egg yolk, nuts, wheat germ.

YOU MAY EAT white rice and pasta, cauliflower, potato, fruits, non iodized salt, drink water.

Date treated:_____ Cleared:_____

Combinations needed:.. A/...B/...D/...R/...H/...C/...N/...N+A/...N+B/...N+H/...N+C/... N+A+H/...N+B+H/...N+A+C/...N+B+C/...EB/...EB+A/...EB+B/...EB+N/...
EB+H/...EB+C/...EB+N+A/...EB+N+B/...EB+N+A+H/...EB+N+B+H/.... EB+N+A+C/... EB+N+B+C/.....

Symptoms Noted:_____
Notes:_____
_____

52. MOLYBDENUM

AVOID whole grains, brown rice, brewers yeast, legumes, buckwheat, millet, dark green leafy vegetables.

YOU MAY EAT white rice and pasta, cauliflower, potato, fresh fruits, non iodized salt, drink water.

Date treated:_____ Cleared:_____

Combinations needed:....................... A/.....B/.....D/.....R/.....H/.......C/.....N/.....N+A/.......N+B/.....N+H/.....N+C/.....N+A+H/.....N+B+H/.....N+A+C/.....N+B+C/.....EB/.....EB+A/.....EB+B/.....EB+N/.....EB+H/ ...EB+C/ ..... +N+A/....EB+N+B/... EB+N+A+H/.... EB+N+B+H/.... EB+N+A+C/ ...EB+N+B+C/.....

Symptoms Noted:_____
Notes:_____
_____

53. PHOSPHORUS

AVOID whole grains, seeds, nuts, legumes, dairy products, egg yolks, fish, corn, dried fruits, poultry and meat.

YOU MAY EAT steamed white rice, potato, cauliflower, fresh fruit, fresh vegetable and vegetable oil.

Date treated:_____ Cleared: _____

Combinations needed:.. A/...B/...D/...R/...H/...C/...N/...N+A/...N+B/...N+H/...N+C/... N+A+H/...N+B+H/...N+A+C/...N+B+C/...EB/...EB+A/...EB+B/...EB+N/...
EB+H/...EB+C/...EB+N+A/...EB+N+B/...EB+N+A+H/...EB+N+B+H/.... EB+N+A+C/... EB+N+B+C/.....

Symptoms Noted:_____

Notes:_____
_____

54. POTASSIUM

AVOID all vegetables, oranges, bananas, cantaloupe, tomatoes, mint leaves, water cress, potatoes, whole grains, seeds, nuts, and cream of tartar.

YOU MAY EAT white rice and pasta, cauliflower, chicken, meat, eggs.

Date treated:_____ Cleared: _____

Combinations needed:.. A/...B/...D/...R/...H/...C/...N/...N+A/...N+B/...N+H/...N+C/... N+A+H/...N+B+H/...N+A+C/...N+B+C/...EB/...EB+A/...EB+B/...EB+N/...
EB+H/...EB+C/...EB+N+A/...EB+N+B/...EB+N+A+H/...EB+N+B+H/.... EB+N+A+C/... EB+N+B+C/.....

Symptoms Noted:_____

Notes:_____
_____

55. SELENIUM

AVOID brewers yeast, wheat germ, kelp, sea water, sea salt, garlic, mushrooms, sea food, milk, eggs, whole grains, beef, beans, bran, onions, tomato, broccoli.

YOU MAY EAT white rice and pasta, cauliflower, potato, chicken, fruits, table salt, drink water.

Date treated:_____   Cleared:_____

Combinations needed:.. A/...B/...D/...R/...H/...C/...N/...N+A/...N+B/...N+H/...N+C/... N+A+H/...N+B+H/...N+A+C/...N+B+C/...EB/...EB+A/...EB+B/...EB+N/...
EB+H/...EB+C/...EB+N+A/...EB+N+B/...EB+N+A+H/...EB+N+B+H/.... EB+N+A+C/... EB+N+B+C/.....

Symptoms Noted:_____
Notes:_____
_____

56. SULPHUR

AVOID radish, turnip, onion, celery, string beans, watercress, soybean, fish, meat, dried beans, eggs, cabbage.

YOU MAY EAT: white rice and pasta, cauliflower, potato, fruits, non iodized salt, drinking water.

Date treated:_____   Cleared:_____

Combinations needed:.. A/...B/...D/...R/...H/...C/...N/...N+A/...N+B/...N+H/...N+C/... N+A+H/...N+B+H/...N+A+C/...N+B+C/...EB/...EB+A/...EB+B/...EB+N/...
EB+H/...EB+C/...EB+N+A/...EB+N+B/...EB+N+A+H/...EB+N+B+H/.... EB+N+A+C/... EB+N+B+C/.....

Symptoms Noted:_____
Notes:_____
_____

57. VANADIUM

AVOID fish, seafood.

YOU MAY EAT everything that is not seafood.

Date treated:_____   Cleared:_____

Combinations needed:...................................... A/.....B/.....D/.....R/.....H/......C/.....N/
.....N+A/.......N+B/.....N+H/.....N+C/.....N+A+H/.....N+B+H/.....N+A+C/.....N+B+C/.....
EB/.....EB+A/.....EB+B/.....EB+N/.....EB+H/...EB+C/ ..... EB+N+A/....EB+N+B/
....EB+N+A+H/....EB+N+B+H/....EB+N+A+C/...EB+N+B+C/.....

Symptoms Noted:_____
Notes:_____

58. ZINC

AVOID wheat bran, wheat germ, seeds, dried beans, peas, onions, mushrooms, brewers yeast, milk, eggs, oysters, herring, brown rice, fish, lamp, beef, pork, green leafy vegetables, mustard.

YOU MAY EAT white rice and pasta, cauliflower, potato, chicken, table salt, drink water.

Date treated:_____   Cleared:_____

Combinations needed:.. A/...B/...D/...R/...H/...C/...N/...N+A/...N+B/...N+H/...N+C/... N+A+H/...N+B+H/
...N+A+C/...N+B+C/...EB/...EB+A/...EB+B/...EB+N/...EB+H/...EB+C/...EB+N+A/...EB+N+B/
...EB+N+A+H/...EB+N+B+H/.... EB+N+A+C/... EB+N+B+C/

Symptoms Noted:_____
Notes:_____

59. SOYBEAN MIX

AVOID all soy products including soy oil, soy milk, soy curd or tofu.

YOU MAY EAT everything without soybean product.

Date treated:_____ Cleared:_____

Combinations needed:.. A/...B/...D/...R/...H/...C/...N/...N+A/...N+B/...N+H/...N+C/... N+A+H/...N+B+H/...N+A+C/...N+B+C/...EB/...EB+A/...EB+B/...EB+N/...
EB+H/...EB+C/...EB+N+A/...EB+N+B/...EB+N+A+H/...EB+N+B+H/.... EB+N+A+C/... EB+N+B+C/.....

Symptoms Noted:_____
Notes:_____
_____

60. LECITHIN

AVOID lecithin products, including cookies, candy bars, vitamins with lecithin, soy lecithin etc.

YOU MAY EAT white rice, cauliflower, potato, water.

Date treated: _____ Cleared:_____

Combinations needed:.. A/...B/...D/...R/...H/...C/...N/...N+A/...N+B/...N+H/...N+C/... N+A+H/...N+B+H/...N+A+C/...N+B+C/...EB/...EB+A/...EB+B/...EB+N/...
EB+H/...EB+C/...EB+N+A/...EB+N+B/...EB+N+A+H/...EB+N+B+H/.... EB+N+A+C/... EB+N+B+C/.....

Symptoms Noted:_____
Notes:_____
_____

61. MILK MIX: (Cow's milk, goat's milk, breast milk).

AVOID all milk products.

YOU MAY EAT everything without milk.

Date treated: _____ Cleared: _____

Combinations needed:.. A/...B/...D/...R/...H/...C/...N/...N+A/...N+B/...N+H/...N+C/... N+A+H/...N+B+H/...N+A+C/...N+B+C/...EB/...EB+A/...EB+B/...EB+N/...
EB+H/...EB+C/...EB+N+A/...EB+N+B/...EB+N+A+H/...EB+N+B+H/.... EB+N+A+C/... EB+N+B+C/
.....

Symptoms Noted: _____
Notes: _____
_____

62. CHEESE MIX: (American, cheddar, jack, parmesan, mozzarella, cottage).

AVOID all products made from cheese.

YOU MAY EAT everything other than cheese.

Date treated: _____ Cleared: _____

Combinations needed:.. A/...B/...D/...R/...H/...C/...N/...N+A/...N+B/...N+H/...N+C/... N+A+H/...N+B+H/...N+A+C/...N+B+C/...EB/...EB+A/...EB+B/...EB+N/...
EB+H/...EB+C/...EB+N+A/...EB+N+B/...EB+N+A+H/...EB+N+B+H/.... EB+N+A+C/... EB+N+B+C/

Symptoms Noted: _____
Notes: _____
_____

63. <u>TOMATO MIX:</u> (green, yellow, red tomato).

AVOID tomatoes of all kinds, and the products made from tomato.

YOU MAY EAT everything without tomato or it's product.

Date treated: _____ Cleared: _____

Combinations needed:.. A/...B/...D/...R/...H/...C/...N/...N+A/...N+B/...N+H/...N+C/... N+A+H/...N+B+H/...N+A+C/...N+B+C/...EB/...EB+A/...EB+B/...EB+N/...
EB+H/...EB+C/...EB+N+A/...EB+N+B/...EB+N+A+H/...EB+N+B+H/.... EB+N+A+C/... EB+N+B+C/.....

Symptoms Noted:_____
Notes:_____
_____

64. <u>ONION MIX:</u> (brown, red, white, green).

AVOID onions and the products made from onions.

YOU MAY EAT everything except onions.

Date treated: _____ Cleared:_____

Combinations needed:.. A/...B/...D/...R/...H/...C/...N/...N+A/...N+B/...N+H/...N+C/... N+A+H/...N+B+H/...N+A+C/...N+B+C/...EB/...EB+A/...EB+B/...EB+N/...
EB+H/...EB+C/...EB+N+A/...EB+N+B/...EB+N+A+H/...EB+N+B+H/.... EB+N+A+C/... EB+N+B+C/

Symptoms Noted:_____
Notes:_____

65. PEPPER MIX: (red, green, black, yellow, Mexican, Italian, Indian peppers).

AVOID all peppers and anything made from peppers.

YOU MAY EAT anything other peppers.

Date treated: _____ Cleared: _____

Combinations needed:.. A/...B/...D/...R/...H/...C/...N/...N+A/...N+B/...N+H/...N+C/... N+A+H/...N+B+H/...N+A+C/...N+B+C/...EB/...EB+A/...EB+B/...EB+N/...
EB+H/...EB+C/...EB+N+A/...EB+N+B/...EB+N+A+H/...EB+N+B+H/.... EB+N+A+C/... EB+N+B+C/.....

Symptoms Noted:_____
Notes:_____
_____

66. POTATO MIX: (russet, white, red, sweet, yam).

AVOID all type of potatoes and the products made from potato.

YOU MAY EAT anything that does not have potato.

Date treated: _____ Cleared: _____

Combinations needed:.. A/...B/...D/...R/...H/...C/...N/...N+A/...N+B/...N+H/...N+C/... N+A+H/...N+B+H/...N+A+C/...N+B+C/...EB/...EB+A/...EB+B/...EB+N/...
EB+H/...EB+C/...EB+N+A/...EB+N+B/...EB+N+A+H/...EB+N+B+H/.... EB+N+A+C/... EB+N+B+C/.....

Symptoms Noted:_____
Notes:_____
_____

67. WHEAT MIX: (red, buck wheat, white).

AVOID all wheat products.

YOU MAY EAT everything other than wheat products.

Date treated:_____ Cleared: _____

Combinations needed:.. A/...B/...D/...R/...H/...C/...N/...N+A/...N+B/...N+H/...N+C/... N+A+H/...N+B+H/...N+A+C/...N+B+C/...EB/...EB+A/...EB+B/...EB+N/...
EB+H/...EB+C/...EB+N+A/...EB+N+B/...EB+N+A+H/...EB+N+B+H/.... EB+N+A+C/... EB+N+B+C/.....

Symptoms Noted: _____
Notes: _____
_____

68. CUCUMBER MIX: (green, pickled).

AVOID: Cucumber and pickles and products made from cucumber like soaps, salad dressings, face creams etc.

YOU MAY EAT anything that doesn't have cucumber.

Date treated:_____ Cleared: _____

Combinations needed:.. A/...B/...D/...R/...H/...C/...N/...N+A/...N+B/...N+H/...N+C/... N+A+H/...N+B+H/...N+A+C/...N+B+C/...EB/...EB+A/...EB+B/...EB+N/...
EB+H/...EB+C/...EB+N+A/...EB+N+B/...EB+N+A+H/...EB+N+B+H/.... EB+N+A+C/... EB+N+B+C/.....

Symptoms Noted: _____
Notes: _____
_____

69. MELON MIX: (Crenshaw, water, cantaloupe, honey dew, pumpkin).

AVOID all types of melons.

YOU MAY EAT everything else other than melon.

Date treated:_____ Cleared:_____

Combinations needed:.. A/...B/...D/...R/...H/...C/...N/...N+A/...N+B/...N+H/...N+C/... N+A+H/...N+B+H/...N+A+C/...N+B+C/...EB/...EB+A/...EB+B/...EB+N/...
EB+H/...EB+C/...EB+N+A/...EB+N+B/...EB+N+A+H/...EB+N+B+H/.... EB+N+A+C/... EB+N+B+C/

Symptoms Noted:_____

Notes:_____
_____

70. MODIFIED STARCH: (refined starches from Potato, corn, arrow root, rice, all purpose flour).

AVOID all starch products, refined grain products, vitamins, certain prescription drugs (read labels), table salt, thick sauces.

YOU MAY EAT vegetables, meats, eggs, beans.

Date treated:_____ Cleared: _____

Combinations needed:.. A/...B/...D/...R/...H/...C/...N/...N+A/...N+B/...N+H/...N+C/... N+A+H/...N+B+H/...N+A+C/...N+B+C/...EB/...EB+A/...EB+B/...EB+N/...
EB+H/...EB+C/...EB+N+A/...EB+N+B/...EB+N+A+H/...EB+N+B+H/.... EB+N+A+C/... EB+N+B+C/

Symptoms Noted:_____

Notes:_____
_____

ENVIRONMENTAL ALLERGENS

1. PESTICIDES.

AVOID fresh vegetables, fruits, meats, insecticides, new mattress, malathion sprays, ant bates, and house, grass, weeds, lawns, trees that have been sprayed for pesticides.

YOU MAY EAT cooked grains, vegetables and fruits.

Date treated: _____ Cleared: _____

Combinations needed:.. A/...B/...D/...R/...H/...C/...N/...N+A/...N+B/...N+H/...N+C/... N+A+H/...N+B+H/...N+A+C/...N+B+C/...EB/...EB+A/...EB+B/...EB+N/...
EB+H/...EB+C/...EB+N+A/...EB+N+B/...EB+N+A+H/...EB+N+B+H/.... EB+N+A+C/... EB+N+B+C/.....

Symptoms Noted:_____
Notes:_____
_____

2. WOOD MIX

AVOID contact with woods, things made with woods. You may wear a pair of gloves to avoid contacts with wooden surfaces.

Date treated:_____ Cleared: _____

Combinations needed:.. A/...B/...D/...R/...H/...C/...N/...N+A/...N+B/...N+H/...N+C/... N+A+H/...N+B+H/...N+A+C/...N+B+C/...EB/...EB+A/...EB+B/...EB+N/...
EB+H/...EB+C/...EB+N+A/...EB+N+B/...EB+N+A+H/...EB+N+B+H/.... EB+N+A+C/... EB+N+B+C/.....

Symptoms Noted:_____
Notes:_____

3. PERFUME MIX

AVOID perfumed soaps, make-up products, hair sprays, flowers.

You may wear a mask to avoid the smell.

Date treated:_____ Cleared: _____

Combinations needed:.. A/...B/...D/...R/...H/...C/...N/...N+A/...N+B/...N+H/...N+C/... N+A+H/...N+B+H/...N+A+C/...N+B+C/...EB/...EB+A/...EB+B/...EB+N/...
EB+H/...EB+C/...EB+N+A/...EB+N+B/...EB+N+A+H/...EB+N+B+H/.... EB+N+A+C/... EB+N+B+C/.....

Symptoms Noted:_____
Notes:_____
_____

4. SMOKING: (nicotine, tobacco).

AVOID smoking areas, smoke from cigarettes, clothes and substances made contact with cigarette smoke. You may wear a mask for 25 hours.

Date treated:_____ Cleared: _____

Combinations needed:.. A/...B/...D/...R/...H/...C/...N/...N+A/...N+B/...N+H/...N+C/... N+A+H/...N+B+H/...N+A+C/...N+B+C/...EB/...EB+A/...EB+B/...EB+N/...
EB+H/...EB+C/...EB+N+A/...EB+N+B/...EB+N+A+H/...EB+N+B+H/.... EB+N+A+C/... EB+N+B+C/.....

Symptoms Noted:_____
Notes:_____
_____

5. HORMONES (estrogen, progesterone, testosterone).

AVOID eating or using red meats and products with hormones. If one is able to get the meat from an animal that has never received any hormone, it is OK to eat the red meat from that source. Avoid stimulating your own hormones. Avoid treating during menstrual period.

Date treated:_____   Cleared:_____

Combinations needed:.. A/...B/...D/...R/...H/...C/...N/...N+A/...N+B/...N+H/...N+C/... N+A+H/...N+B+H/...N+A+C/...N+B+C/...EB/...EB+A/...EB+B/...EB+N/...
EB+H/...EB+C/...EB+N+A/...EB+N+B/...EB+N+A+H/...EB+N+B+H/.... EB+N+A+C/... EB+N+B+C/.....

Symptoms Noted:_____

Notes:_____
_____

6. BACTERIA MIX: (Strepto-coccus, staphylo-coccus).

AVOID contact with infected surfaces.

YOU MAY EAT everything well cooked and drink boiled, cooled water.

Date treated:_____   Cleared:_____

Combinations needed:.. A/...B/...D/...R/...H/...C/...N/...N+A/...N+B/...N+H/...N+C/... N+A+H/...N+B+H/...N+A+C/...N+B+C/...EB/...EB+A/...EB+B/...EB+N/...
EB+H/...EB+C/...EB+N+A/...EB+N+B/...EB+N+A+H/...EB+N+B+H/.... EB+N+A+C/... EB+N+B+C/.....

Symptoms Noted:_____

Notes:_____
_____

The NAET Guide Book

7. VIRUS MIX: (E.B.V., C.M.V., herpes simplex, herpes zoaster, influenza).

AVOID contact with infected persons for 25 hours. If someone is infected with a virus, treat for the specific sample like herpes zoaster, etc. Also you may take a sample of your own body fluid (saliva, urine, stool, blood, skin tissue, etc.) and treat for it.

YOU MAY EAT everything well cooked and drink boiled, cooled water.

Date treated:_____ Cleared:_____

Combinations needed:.. A/...B/...D/...R/...H/...C/...N/...N+A/...N+B/...N+H/...N+C/... N+A+H/...N+B+H/...N+A+C/...N+B+C/...EB/...EB+A/...EB+B/...EB+N/...
EB+H/...EB+C/...EB+N+A/...EB+N+B/...EB+N+A+H/...EB+N+B+H/.... EB+N+A+C/... EB+N+B+C/.....

Symptoms Noted:_____
Notes:_____
_____

8. CHEMICALS; (soaps, detergents, cleansing chemicals, chlorine, Clorox, bleach).

AVOID contact with the above items for 25 hours. Wash your clothes in plain water prior to treatment.

Date treated:_____ Cleared:_____

Combinations needed:.. A/...B/...D/...R/...H/...C/...N/...N+A/...N+B/...N+H/...N+C/... N+A+H/...N+B+H/...N+A+C/...N+B+C/...EB/...EB+A/...EB+B/...EB+N/...
EB+H/...EB+C/...EB+N+A/...EB+N+B/...EB+N+A+H/...EB+N+B+H/.... EB+N+A+C/... EB+N+B+C/.....

Symptoms Noted:_____
Notes:_____
_____

9. RADIATION: (sun, microwave, T.V., X-ray, computer).

AVOID sun, T.V., microwave, X-ray & computers for 25 hours.

Date treated:_____ Cleared:_____

Combinations needed:.. A/...B/...D/...R/...H/...C/...N/...N+A/...N+B/...N+H/...N+C/... N+A+H/...N+B+H/...N+A+C/...N+B+C/...EB/...EB+A/...EB+B/...EB+N/...

EB+H/...EB+C/...EB+N+A/...EB+N+B/...EB+N+A+H/...EB+N+B+H/.... EB+N+A+C/... EB+N+B+C/.....

Symptoms Noted:_____

Notes:_____
_____

10. FREON

AVOID air conditioned areas, soft plastic products(fluoromethane).

Date treated:_____ Cleared:_____

Combinations needed:.. A/...B/...D/...R/...H/...C/...N/...N+A/...N+B/...N+H/...N+C/... N+A+H/...N+B+H/...N+A+C/...N+B+C/...EB/...EB+A/...EB+B/...EB+N/...

EB+H/...EB+C/...EB+N+A/...EB+N+B/...EB+N+A+H/...EB+N+B+H/.... EB+N+A+C/... EB+N+B+C/.....

Symptoms Noted:_____

Notes:_____
_____

11. POLLEN MIX

AVOID going out doors. wear a mask.

Date treated: _____ Cleared: _____

Combinations needed:.. A/...B/...D/...R/...H/...C/...N/...N+A/...N+B/...N+H/...N+C/... N+A+H/...N+B+H/...N+A+C/...N+B+C/...EB/...EB+A/...EB+B/...EB+N/...

EB+H/...EB+C/...EB+N+A/...EB+N+B/...EB+N+A+H/...EB+N+B+H/.... EB+N+A+C/... EB+N+B+C/

Symptoms Noted:_____

Notes:_____
_____

12. WEED MIX

AVOID going out doors. Wear a mask.

Date treated: _____ Cleared: _____

Combinations needed:.. A/...B/...D/...R/...H/...C/...N/...N+A/...N+B/...N+H/...N+C/... N+A+H/...N+B+H/...N+A+C/...N+B+C/...EB/...EB+A/...EB+B/...EB+N/...

EB+H/...EB+C/...EB+N+A/...EB+N+B/...EB+N+A+H/...EB+N+B+H/.... EB+N+A+C/... EB+N+B+C/
.....

Symptoms Noted:_____

Notes:_____
_____

13. GRASS MIX

AVOID going out doors. Wear shoes and socks while walking outside.

Date treated:_____ Cleared: _____

Combinations needed:.. A/...B/...D/...R/...H/...C/...N/...N+A/...N+B/...N+H/...N+C/... N+A+H/...N+B+H/...N+A+C/...N+B+C/...EB/...EB+A/...EB+B/...EB+N/...

EB+H/...EB+C/...EB+N+A/...EB+N+B/...EB+N+A+H/...EB+N+B+H/.... EB+N+A+C/... EB+N+B+C/.....

Symptoms Noted:_____

Notes:_____

_____

14. TREE MIX

AVOID going outdoors. Wear shoes and socks while walking outside. Wear mask and gloves if you are going out.

Date treated:_____ Cleared: _____

Combinations needed:.. A/...B/...D/...R/...H/...C/...N/...N+A/...N+B/...N+H/...N+C/... N+A+H/...N+B+H/...N+A+C/...N+B+C/...EB/...EB+A/...EB+B/...EB+N/...

EB+H/...EB+C/...EB+N+A/...EB+N+B/...EB+N+A+H/...EB+N+B+H/.... EB+N+A+C/... EB+N+B+C/

Symptoms Noted:_____

Notes:_____

_____

15. DUST MIX and dust mites.

AVOID dusty areas. Clean up the living area before the treatment. Wear a mask for 25 hours.

Date treated:_____ Cleared: _____

Combinations needed:.. A/...B/...D/...R/...H/...C/...N/...N+A/...N+B/...N+H/...N+C/... N+A+H/...N+B+H/...N+A+C/...N+B+C/...EB/...EB+A/...EB+B/...EB+N/...
EB+H/...EB+C/...EB+N+A/...EB+N+B/...EB+N+A+H/...EB+N+B+H/.... EB+N+A+C/... EB+N+B+C/.....

Symptoms Noted:_____
Notes:_____
_____

16. MOLD MIX

AVOID treating on a cloudy, rainy day. Clean up the house well. Keep the house dry. Stay away from leaky bathrooms, old houses, etc. Wear freshly washed clothes.

Date treated:_____ Cleared: _____

Combinations needed:.. A/...B/...D/...R/...H/...C/...N/...N+A/...N+B/...N+H/...N+C/... N+A+H/...N+B+H/...N+A+C/...N+B+C/...EB/...EB+A/...EB+B/...EB+N/...
EB+H/...EB+C/...EB+N+A/...EB+N+B/...EB+N+A+H/...EB+N+B+H/.... EB+N+A+C/... EB+N+B+C/.....

Symptoms Noted:_____
Notes:_____
_____

17. MERCURY MIX/AMALGAM

AVOID fish and fish products. avoid mercury products. avoid touching your mouth if you have dental fillings. Wear a pair of gloves for 25 hours.

Date treated:_____ Cleared :_____

Combinations needed:.. A/...B/...D/...R/...H/...C/...N/...N+A/...N+B/...N+H/...N+C/... N+A+H/...N+B+H/...N+A+C/...N+B+C/...EB/...EB+A/...EB+B/...EB+N/...

EB+H/...EB+C/...EB+N+A/...EB+N+B/...EB+N+A+H/...EB+N+B+H/.... EB+N+A+C/... EB+N+B+C/.....

Symptoms Noted:_____
Notes:_____
_____

18. NEWSPAPER products.

AVOID touching paper goods, newspaper, facial paper, hand towel, pine products, tissue paper etc.

Date treated:_____ Cleared:_____

Combinations needed:.. A/...B/...D/...R/...H/...C/...N/...N+A/...N+B/...N+H/...N+C/... N+A+H/...N+B+H/...N+A+C/...N+B+C/...EB/...EB+A/...EB+B/...EB+N/...EB+H/...EB+C/...EB+N+A/...EB+N+B/...EB+N+A+H/...EB+N+B+H/.... EB+N+A+C/... EB+N+B+C/.....

Symptoms Noted:_____
Notes:_____
_____

19. INSECT MIX: (Bee, ant, spider, flea).

AVOID touching or going near any insects.

Date treated:_____ Cleared:_____

Combinations needed:.. A/...B/...D/...R/...H/...C/...N/...N+A/...N+B/...N+H/...N+C/... N+A+H/...N+B+H/...N+A+C/...N+B+C/...EB/...EB+A/...EB+B/...EB+N/...
EB+H/...EB+C/...EB+N+A/...EB+N+B/...EB+N+A+H/...EB+N+B+H/.... EB+N+A+C/... EB+N+B+C/

Symptoms Noted:_____
Notes:_____
_____

20. FABRIC MIX

Try to treat one kind of fabric first, like cotton or polyester, etc. Then wear the allergy-cleared item while treating for the fabric mix.

AVOID contact with the fabric that is being treated.

Date treated:_____ Cleared:_____

Combinations needed:.. A/...B/...D/...R/...H/...C/...N/...N+A/...N+B/...N+H/...N+C/... N+A+H/...N+B+H/...N+A+C/...N+B+C/...EB/...EB+A/...EB+B/...EB+N/...
EB+H/...EB+C/...EB+N+A/...EB+N+B/...EB+N+A+H/...EB+N+B+H/.... EB+N+A+C/... EB+N+B+C/

Symptoms Noted:_____
Notes:_____
_____

21. ANIMAL EPITHELIAL/DANDER.

AVOID contact with the animals, their saliva, hair, danders, any other products made from animals or used by the animals. If you have a pet, make arrangements to stay away from him/her for 25 hours.

Date treated:_____ Cleared: _____

Combinations needed:.. A/...B/...D/...R/...H/...C/...N/...N+A/...N+B/...N+H/...N+C/... N+A+H/...N+B+H/...N+A+C/...N+B+C/...EB/...EB+A/...EB+B/...EB+N/...
EB+H/...EB+C/...EB+N+A/...EB+N+B/...EB+N+A+H/...EB+N+B+H/.... EB+N+A+C/... EB+N+B+C/.....

Symptoms Noted:_____

Notes:_____
_____

22. FORMALDEHYDE

AVOID new buildings, new clothes, newspaper, liquid paper, pressed woods,
paints, paint thinners, fumes, perfumes, certain ice creams. Wear a mask and use a pair of gloves.

Date treated:_____ Cleared: _____

Combinations needed:.. A/...B/...D/...R/...H/...C/...N/...N+A/...N+B/...N+H/...N+C/... N+A+H/...N+B+H/...N+A+C/...N+B+C/...EB/...EB+A/...EB+B/...EB+N/...
EB+H/...EB+C/...EB+N+A/...EB+N+B/...EB+N+A+H/...EB+N+B+H/.... EB+N+A+C/... EB+N+B+C/.....

Symptoms Noted:_____
Notes:_____

23. PLASTICS

AVOID all plastic and crude oil products including computer key boards, telephones, pens, vinyl chairs, containers, book covers, toothbrush, hair brush etc.

Date treated:_____ Cleared:_____ _____

Combinations needed:.. A/...B/...D/...R/...H/...C/...N/...N+A/...N+B/...N+H/...N+C/... N+A+H/...N+B+H/...N+A+C/...N+B+C/...EB/...EB+A/...EB+B/...EB+N/...
EB+H/...EB+C/...EB+N+A/...EB+N+B/...EB+N+A+H/...EB+N+B+H/.... EB+N+A+C/... EB+N+B+C/.....

Symptoms Noted:_____
Notes:_____
_____

24. PARASITE MIX: (Pin worm, tape worm, hook worm, amoeba, giardia, protozoa)

AVOID eating anything uncooked. Drink boiled water.

Date treated:_____ Cleared:_____

Combinations needed:.. A/...B/...D/...R/...H/...C/...N/...N+A/...N+B/...N+H/...N+C/... N+A+H/...N+B+H/...N+A+C/...N+B+C/...EB/...EB+A/...EB+B/...EB+N/...
EB+H/...EB+C/...EB+N+A/...EB+N+B/...EB+N+A+H/...EB+N+B+H/.... EB+N+A+C/... EB+N+B+C/.....

Symptoms Noted:_____
Notes:_____
_____

ITEM TREATED:_____
AVOID:_____
Date treated:_____ Cleared:_____

Combinations needed:................................. A/.....B/.....D/.....R/.....H/......C/
.....N/..
...N+A/......N+B/.....N+H/.....N+C/.....N+A+H/.....N+B+H/.....N+A+C/.....N+B+C/.....
EB/.....EB+A/.....EB+B/.....EB+N/.....EB+H/ ...EB+C/ ..... EB+N+A/....EB+N+B/..
..EB+N+A+H/....EB+N+B+H/....EB+N+A+C/...EB+N+B+C/.....

Symptoms Noted: _____

Notes: _____
_____

ITEM TREATED: _____

AVOID: _____

Date treated: _____ Cleared: _____

Combinations needed:.. A/...B/...D/...R/...H/...C/...N/...N+A/...N+B/...N+H/...N+C/... N+A+H/...N+B+H/
...N+A+C/...N+B+C/...EB/...EB+A/...EB+B/...EB+N/...

EB+H/...EB+C/...EB+N+A/...EB+N+B/...EB+N+A+H/...EB+N+B+H/.... EB+N+A+C/... EB+N+B+C/
.....

Symptoms Noted: _____

Notes: _____
_____

ITEM TREATED: _____

AVOID: _____

Date treated: _____ Cleared: _____

Combinations needed:.. A/...B/...D/...R/...H/...C/...N/...N+A/...N+B/...N+H/...N+C/... N+A+H/...N+B+H/
...N+A+C/...N+B+C/...EB/...EB+A/...EB+B/...EB+N/...

EB+H/...EB+C/...EB+N+A/...EB+N+B/...EB+N+A+H/...EB+N+B+H/.... EB+N+A+C/... EB+N+B+C/
.....

Symptoms Noted: _____

Notes: _____
_____

ITEM TREATED: _____

AVOID: _____

Date treated: _____ Cleared: _____

Combinations needed:.. A/...B/...D/...R/...H/...C/...N/...N+A/...N+B/...N+H/...N+C/... N+A+H/...N+B+H/
...N+A+C/...N+B+C/...EB/...EB+A/...EB+B/...EB+N/...

EB+H/...EB+C/...EB+N+A/...EB+N+B/...EB+N+A+H/...EB+N+B+H/.... EB+N+A+C/... EB+N+B+C/

Symptoms Noted: _____

Notes: _____

_____

ITEM TREATED: _____

AVOID: _____

Date treated: _____ Cleared: _____

Combinations needed:.. A/...B/...D/...R/...H/...C/...N/...N+A/...N+B/...N+H/...N+C/... N+A+H/...N+B+H/...N+A+C/...N+B+C/...EB/...EB+A/...EB+B/...EB+N/...

EB+H/...EB+C/...EB+N+A/...EB+N+B/...EB+N+A+H/...EB+N+B+H/.... EB+N+A+C/... EB+N+B+C/.....

Symptoms Noted: _____

Notes: _____

_____

ITEM TREATED: _____

AVOID _____

Combinations needed:.. A/...B/...D/...R/...H/...C/...N/...N+A/...N+B/...N+H/...N+C/... N+A+H/...N+B+H/...N+A+C/...N+B+C/...EB/...EB+A/...EB+B/...EB+N/...

EB+H/...EB+C/...EB+N+A/...EB+N+B/...EB+N+A+H/...EB+N+B+H/.... EB+N+A+C/... EB+N+B+C/.....

Symptoms Noted: _____

Notes: _____

_____

ITEM TREATED: _____

AVOID: _____

Date treated: _____ Cleared: _____

Combinations needed:.. A/...B/...D/...R/...H/...C/...N/...N+A/...N+B/...N+H/...N+C/... N+A+H/...N+B+H/...N+A+C/...N+B+C/...EB/...EB+A/...EB+B/...EB+N/...

EB+H/...EB+C/...EB+N+A/...EB+N+B/...EB+N+A+H/...EB+N+B+H/.... EB+N+A+C/... EB+N+B+C/.....

Symptoms Noted: _____

Notes: _____

_____

ITEM TREATED: _____

AVOID: _____

Date treated: _____ Cleared: _____

Combinations needed:.. A/...B/...D/...R/...H/...C/...N/...N+A/...N+B/...N+H/...N+C/... N+A+H/...N+B+H/...N+A+C/...N+B+C/...EB/...EB+A/...EB+B/...EB+N/...

EB+H/...EB+C/...EB+N+A/...EB+N+B/...EB+N+A+H/...EB+N+B+H/.... EB+N+A+C/... EB+N+B+C/.....

Symptoms Noted: _____

Notes: _____

_____

RESOURCES FOR HEALTH PRODUCTS

Lotus Herbs, Inc.
1124 N. Hacienda Blvd.
La Puente, CA 91744
(818) 916-1070
(Chinese heral formula)

Neuro Emotional Techniques
Dr. Scott Walker
524, 2nd Street,
Encinitas, CA 92024

La Chance Release Method
Dr. Toby Campion, D.C.
8818 W. Olympic Blvd.
Bevery Hills, CA 90211
(310) 273-1221

Kenshin trading Corp.
1815 W. 213th St., #180
Torrance, CA 90501
(310) 212-3199
(Nutritional Products - Garlic, Kelp, Sanza)

Integris Inc.
11 Daytona
Laguna Niguel, CA 92677
(714) 363-9822.
Contact: Dr. David Nelson.
(Nutritional Supplements).

Standard Process Lab.
5621 Palmer Way, Ste.F
Carlsbad, CA 92008
(800) 372-7218
(Nutritional Supplements).

Thorne Research
901 Triangle Dr.,
Sandpoint, ID 83864
(208) 263-1337
(Nutritional Supplements).

Allergy Research
400 Preda Street,
San Leandro, CA 94577.
(800)782-4274

Metagenics, Inc.
971 Calle Negocio
San Clemente,
CA 92673
(714) 366-0818

Chiro-Tech, Inc.
628 Calle Plano
Camarillo, CA 93010
(805) 388-7127
(Air Purifiers).

Digital Health
1225 E. Fort Union Blvd., Ste. #200
Midvale, UT 84047-1882
(801) 561-4707

CFIDS Buyers Club
1187 Coast Village Road, #1280
Santa Barbara, CA 93108
(800) 366- 6056

Herb Finders
P.O.BOx 3868
Salt Lake City, UT 84110
(800) 780-6934
(Turkey Rhubarb Formula)

Vitamin Shoppe
4700 Westside Ave.
NewJersey, NJ 07047
(800) 223-1216
(Colloidal Mineral Complex).

Lab Testing
Great Smoky Mountain Lab
18 A Regent Park Blvd.
Ashville, NC 28806
(800)522-4762

Janice Corp.
198 US High Way 46
Budd Lake, NJ 07828-3001
(800) 526-4237
(Cotton Gloves)

Delta Publishing Co.
6714 Beach Blvd.
Buena Park, CA 90621
Tel. (714) 523-0800
Fax: (714) 523-3068
{ Say Goodbye To Illness}
{Living Pain Free}
Web site: allergy-naet.com

BIBLIOGRAPHY

ESSENTIALS OF CHINESE ACUPUNCTURE compiled by Beijing College of traditional Chinese Medicine, Shanghai College of Traditional Chinese Medicine, Nanjing College of Traditional Chinese Medicine, The Acupuncture Institute of the Academy of Traditional Chinese Medicine, Beijing, China: Foreign Language Press, 1981 (First Edition)

A PHYSICIAN'S HANDBOOK ON ORTHOMOLECULAR MEDICINE ed. by R. J. Williams and D. K. Kalita, Pergamon Press, New York, 1977

NUTRITIONAL SUPPORT OF MEDICAL PRACTICE ed. H.A. Schnelder, C.E. Anderson and D.B. Coursin, Harper & Row Publishers, New York, 1977

MENTAL AND ELEMENTAL NUTRIENTS c. c. Pfeiffer, Keats Publishing, Inc., New Canan, Connecticut, 1975

TRACE ELEMENTS IN HUMAN HEALTH AND DISEASE Vol. 1, "Zinc & Copper" and Vol. 11, "Essential & Toxic Elements," ed. by A. S. Prasad, Academic Press, New York, 1976

FOOD, NUTRITION AND DIET THERAPY M. V. Krause and L. K. Mahan, W. B. Saunders Company, Philadelphia, 1979

EVALUATION OF PROTEINS FOR HUMANS ed. by C. E. Bodwell, AVI Publishing Company, Inc., Westpoint, Connecticut, 1977

SAY GOODBYE TO ILLNESS by D. S. Nambudripad, Delta Publishing Co., Buena Park, CA, First edition 1973, second edition 1998

LIVING PAIN FREE by D. S. Nambudripad, Delta Publishing Co., Buena Park, CA, 1997

YOU CAN REPROGRAM YOUR BRAIN TO PERFECT HEALTH by D. S. Nambudripad, Singer Publishing, Rancho Mirage, CA, 1989

FREEDOM FROM ALLERGIES by D. S. Nambudripad, Delta Publishing Co. Buena Park, CA., 1987

Index

A

Acupuncture 24
Air-conditioning 10
Alcoholism 8
Amalgum 79
Amino Acids 45
Anaphylaxis 19
Animal Fat 44
Arthritis 12
Atmospheric Changes 9
Auto-immune Disorders 12

B

B-complex 34
Bacteria 12
Bacteria Mix 73
Baking Powder 51
Base 56
Basic Treatments 13
Biotin 36
Bleach 74
Blood Disoders 12
Body Movements 11
Buddy System 2
Building Materials 9

C

C.M.V. 74
Calcium Mix 33
Cancer 12
Ceramic Cups 9
Ceramics 9
Cheese Mix 66
Chemicals 9, 74
Chicken 32
Chlorine 74
Chlorox 74
Choline: 36
Chromium 58
Chronic Fatigue 12
Clearing Practitioner's Allergies 2
Clinic Rules 26
Cobalt 58
Coffee Brewing 9
Coffee Mix 41, 42
Cold 9

Combination Treatments 22
Concrete 9
Concrete Floors 9
Copper 59
Corn Mix 40
Cucumber Mix 69

D

Daily Log 6
Dancing 11
Depression 11
Detergents 75
Diabetes 11
Diet 24
Doctor's Office 1
Dried Beans Mix 48
Driveways 9
Driving 11
Dryness 10
Dust Mix 78

E

E.b.v 74
Eating Refined Food 20
Egg Mix. 32
Egg White 32
Egg Yolk 32
Emotional Allergy 23
Emotional Symptoms 4
Environmental Allergens 71
Estrogen 73
Exercise 11, 24

F

Fabric Mix 80
Fabrics 9
Feather 32
Fibromyalgia 12
Fish Mix 46
Flowers 9
Fluoride 50
Folic Acid 36
Food Additives 57

Food Coloring 57
Food Craving 20
Formaldehyde 81
Formaldehyde 9
Freon 75
Frequency of the Treatments 16

G

Gelatin 50
Germanium 59
Gluten Allergy 11
Good Eating Habits 23
Grain Mix 40
Grass Mix 77
Group 1. 5
Group 2. 5
Group 3. 5
Group 4. 5
Group 5. 6
Gum Mix 51

H

Hair Products 9
Heat 9
Herpes 74
High Altitude 10
High Platelets 12
Humidity 9

I

Influenza 74
Inositol 36
Insect Mix 80
Intestinal Disorders 11
Iodine 60
Iron Mix 38
Items To Treat Together 31

J

Jogging 11
Juice Fast 20

L

La Chance Release Techniques 6

Lecithin 65
Leukemia 12
Living Pain Free With Acupressure 12
Lotus Herbs, 6
Low Altitude 10
Low White Blood Cells 12

M

Magnesium 60
Manganese 61
Marbles 9
Massage 24
Melon Mix 70
Mercury 79
Milk Mix 66
Mineral Mix 39
Modified Starch 70
Mold Mix 79
Molybdenum 61
MRT 2

N

NARF 2
NAET 1
Nail Polish 9
Nambudripad's Allergy Elimination Techniques 1
Nambudripad's Allergy Research Foundation 2
Neuro Emotional Techniques 6
Newspaper 9, 79
Normal Reaction after Treatments 3
Nut Mix 1 42
Nut Mix 2 42

O

Onion Mix 67
Order of Treatments 14

P

PABA: 37
Paints 9
Paper 79
Parasites 12
Pepper Mix 68
Perfume Mix 72
Pesticides 71

Phosphorus 62
Physical Symptoms 4
Pollen Mix 76
Popcorn 9
Potassium 62
Potato Mix 68
Preparation for Treatments 12
Progesterone 73

R

Radiation 75
Reactions During Naet 5
RNA/DNA 55
Rowing 11
Running 11

S

Sailing 11
Salt Mix 39
Say Goodbye to Illness 1
Selenium 63
Shellfish Mix 46
Smoking 72
Soaps 74
Soybean 65
Spice Mix 1 43
Spice Mix 2 43
Stomach Acids 56
Sugar Mix 37
Sulphur 63
Supplements 20
Support Group 3
Surrogate Treatment 7

T

Tennis, 11
Testosterone 73
Tetracycline 32
Tiles 9
Tomato Mix 67
Treating for Clouds 10
Tree Mix 77
Turkey 49

U

Unusual Conditions 25

V

Vanadium 64
Vegetable Fats 45
Virus 12
Virus Mix 74
Vitamin B1 34
Vitamin B2 34
Vitamin B3 34
Vitamin A Mix 38
Vitamin B12 35
Vitamin B13 35
Vitamin B15 35
Vitamin B17 35
Vitamin B4 35
Vitamin B5: 35
Vitamin B6 35
Vitamin C Mix 33
Vitamin D 53
Vitamin F 54
Vitamin K 53
Vitamin P 54
Vitamin T 55
vitamin E 52

W

Walking 11
Weakness of the Knees 9
Weed Mix 76
Wheat Mix 69
Whey 47
Whiten-all 49
Wood Furniture 9
Wood Mix 71
Wood Work 9

Y

Yeast Mix 47
Yeast/ Candida 11
Yogurt 48

Z

Zinc 64

Notes